TEN LIES ABOUT AIDS

Etienne de Harven, M.D.

Jean-Claude Roussez

Order this book online at www.trafford.com
or email orders@trafford.com

Most Trafford titles are also available at major online book retailers.

© Copyright 2008 Etienne De Harven, M.D. & Jean-Claude Roussez.
All rights reserved. No part of this publication may be reproduced, stored in a retrieval system, or transmitted, in any form or by any means, electronic, mechanical, photocopying, recording, or otherwise, without the written prior permission of the author.

Print information available on the last page.

ISBN: 978-1-4251-5426-4 (sc)

Because of the dynamic nature of the Internet, any web addresses or links contained in this book may have changed since publication and may no longer be valid. The views expressed in this work are solely those of the author and do not necessarily reflect the views of the publisher, and the publisher hereby disclaims any responsibility for them.

Any people depicted in stock imagery provided by Getty Images are models, and such images are being used for illustrative purposes only.
Certain stock imagery © Getty Images.

Trafford rev. 01/06/2020

Trafford PUBLISHING® www.trafford.com
North America & international
toll-free: 1 888 232 4444 (USA & Canada)
fax: 812 355 4082

TABLE OF CONTENTS

Acknowledgments 9

Foreword 11

Introduction 15

LIE #1   Aids is a new Illness 19

LIE #2   There is an AIDS virus: HIV 25

LIE #3   HIV is the cause of AIDS 41

LIE #4   Antiviral medication is beneficial 51

LIE #5   HIV-positivity is a sign of HIV infection 63

LIE #6   AIDS is contagious 77

LIE #7   HIV causes numerous illnesses 89

LIE #8   It's better to know that you are HIV-positive 101

LIE #9   The AIDS epidemic is overwhelming 107

LIE #10 The scientists all agree 127

Enough Lies 137

Happily, We Have Internet! 143

Epilogue 149

References 153

DEDICATED to the memory of our friend MARK GRIFFITHS, whose wisdom, courage and intellectual integrity have been a source of inspiration for all those who had the good fortune and pleasure of knowing him.

TEN LIES ABOUT AIDS

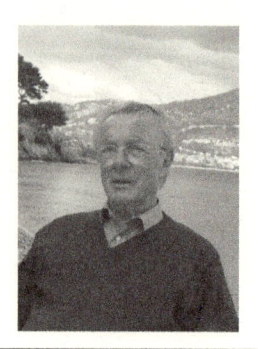

ABOUT THE AUTHOR
ETIENNE DE HARVEN

After obtaining his M.D. degree in 1953 from the Université Libre de Bruxelles, (where he later became *"Professeur Agrégé"* in Pathology), Etienne de Harven specialized in electron microscopy at the "Institut du Cancer" in Paris.

In 1956, he joined Charlotte Friend's team at the Sloan Kettering Institute in New York, the largest cancer research center in the United States, where he was in charge of electron microscopy research. It was there that he produced the world's first description of a retrovirus budding on the surface of infected cells.

In 1981, he was appointed Professor of Pathology and laboratory director at the University of Toronto, Canada, where he researched the marking of antigens on the surface of lymphocytes.

Now retired, he is the President of *Rethinking Aids*, a group comprising over 2000 scientists and other re-thinkers who refute the viral origin of AIDS.

He is also a member of the South African President Thabo Mbeki's International AIDS Advisory Panel.

ETIENNE DE HARVEN, M.D. & JEAN-CLAUDE ROUSSEZ

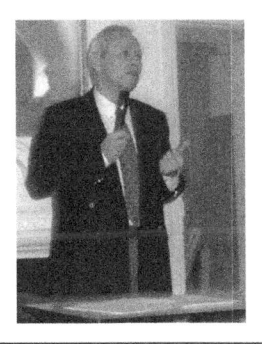

ABOUT THE AUTHOR
JEAN-CLAUDE ROUSSEZ

After advanced studies in electronics, Jean-Claude Roussez entered scientific and technical journalism.

He was editorial Director of the monthly *Radio Plans/ Électronique Loisirs*, and later became the founder and Editor-in-Chief of the professional review *Electronique Applications*, one of whose main focuses was medical electronics.

He published numerous studies related to the application of high technology in medicine, as well as a large number of articles disagreeing with official science.

He is the creator and author of the famous online game "Electronique 2000", and has taken part in some fifty programs popularizing science for young people on the French TV channel TF1.

ABOUT THE COVER

The cover: The folded red ribbon has been a symbol of HIV/AIDS for many years. Obviously, the HIV dogma became highly questionable. The cover page of this book is showing ten cracks in the red ribbon, symbolizing the "Ten lies about AIDS" analysed in this book.

The cover artwork has been designed by Colin Downes-Grainger of London UK www.actionminddrugs.org.uk to whom the authors express their most appreciative thanks.

ACKNOWLEDGMENTS

This book was originally published in French, Dangles editors, 2005, under the title "Les Dix Plus Gros Mensonges sur le Sida". This original version had been carefully reviewed by Dr. Marc Deru, from Belgium.

Dangles Editors kindly gave permission to prepare the present English translation that include only minor alterations by comparison with the original French version.

The authors wish to express their thanks to Susie Kelly who did the first draft of the translation. They also express their gratitude to Anthony Brink, South Africa, for his expert review of the translation and for having kindly accepted writing the Foreword, and to Jan Spreen for his ultimate corrections.

They also wish to express their gratitude to two distinguished friends, involved in the HIV/AIDS debate for many years, and whose generosity made the publication of this English edition possible.

FOREWORD

On 28 February 2000, four months to the day after rocking the AIDS establishment by ordering an enquiry into the safety of the AIDS drug AZT, South African President Thabo Mbeki made known his plans to convene a symposium of orthodox and dissident scientists and clinicians to thrash out the scientific controversy about AIDS and its treatment with AZT and similar drugs.

Most significant was whom President Mbeki personally picked to attend the two meetings of his International AIDS Advisory Panel. What his invitations showed was that he knew exactly who the leading critics of the HIV theory of AIDS were, including the radicals, namely the scientists and doctors – among them one the co-authors of this book, Professor Etienne de Harven – who contend that the HIV theory of AIDS is wrong for the most basic reason: the so-called virus has never been isolated directly from any AIDS patient. And in the Age of AIDS, the President of South Africa is onto this ultimate heresy.

In a public debate in May 2001 with Dr Jerry Coovadia, Professor of HIV-AIDS Research at the University of KwaZulu-Natal, I opened my case by saying: "I've been thinking very deeply about and have been politically engaged with the problem of AIDS for several years now; and I have come to the conclusion that there will never be a resolution of the problem of AIDS until there's been a resolution of the problem of HIV."

And I think this still, because HIV-AIDS is a mythology supporting a vast commercial and professional industry, and for as long people think there's a virus out there being spread during sex, by exposure to blood, and by mothers to their babies, the myth will retain its power over the popular imagination and will remain impervious to refutation by fact and reason, no matter how cogent. This is how faith in gods and demons works. They have to be killed off by being expelled from mass consciousness; and it won't do to merely contend that they're not really as powerful as claimed.This is what makes this important book different from others that have preceded it in laying bare the myths of AIDS. In plain language intelligible to any reader, Etienne de Harven and science journalist Jean-Claude Roussez make the point that in the trial of HIV, charged with causing AIDS, the accused's dock stands empty: the very existence of the accused culprit is an error, even if the legendary figure in everyone's mind has been given a most impressive name by the police and in the newspapers to match the suspicion about him, and various ambiguous clues to the presence of the accused are excitedly deposed to.

To return to the real: De Harven and Roussez make clear that so-called "molecular markers" for "HIV" can never be an acceptable substitute for electron microscope images of retroviral particles, images that are deceptively missing from most of the HIV/AIDS literature.

Notwithstanding its startling and almost unimaginably radical point of departure, this book can't simply be dismissed as any sort of unhinged raving, because Etienne de Harven is a medical scientist of the highest rank and a widely published pioneering expert in the electron microscopy of viruses, no less. And in these matters no one sensible can say he doesn't know what he's talking about.

I met Etienne de Harven at the first meeting of President Mbeki's International AIDS Advisory Panel in May 2000, and since then I have counted him amongst my dearest friends; and

FOREWORD

no trip to Europe is satisfactory without at least two lunches together.

I must say though – to echo 1993 Chemistry Nobel Laureate Dr Kary Mullis's disclaimer in his foreword to Professor Peter Duesberg's *Inventing the AIDS Virus* – that Etienne and I do not see eye to eye on everything written in this book. This is because, since running into the trouble with the HIV theory of AIDS eleven years ago, a great more than just "HIV" has gone up in smoke for me: I'm referring to the very fundamentals of infectious disease theory generally (here Etienne throws up his hands and says, "But I'm a classical pathologist!").

That said, if you still think you can die in about ten years time from making love with your new sweetie, and that drinking deadly poison every day until you die will keep you well if some doctor with a long face tells you that you've got the virus in you because you did, or will keep you alive and make you live longer if for some reason you're sick, here's a book to fix your unfortunate mistakes.

ANTHONY BRINK

Anthony Brink is an advocate of the High Court of South Africa, in Cape Town, and the founder and chairman of the Treatment Information Group.

INTRODUCTION

"An error can never become true however many times you repeat it. The truth can never be wrong, even if no one hears it."
Mahatma Gandhi.

If ever there was a world where fables are currency, it's that of health, and the reason for that is the multitude of opportunities they generate. It stretches from the lowest material greed to the highest level of world politics, perpetuating old mistakes which continue to be claimed as well-founded, despite the lack of evidence based medicine.

Official science has created a dense smokescreen around subjects such as cancers, vaccines, so-called "emergent" infectious illnesses and genetic mutations.

Any study that jeopardizes the huge structure that has been built over more than a century by generations of "mandarins" is either publicly derided, or else interpreted in such a way that it gives birth to theories even more absurd than the previous ones.

Today, scientific deceit is still rife, and its spread is accelerated by the sensation-hungry media. Sadly, those who have the desire and courage to seek the truth, and by doing so debunk the mistakes of science, are very few in number.

A doctor or researcher needs a certain degree of heroism to dare to question universally accepted theories, for by doing so he risks being banished from the scientific community.

Being struck off as a doctor or pharmacist; banned from practicing; legal actions leading to arrest or imprisonment; administrative harassment, withdrawal of research grants, and worse still: this is the lot of those who dare to challenge some aspects of deep-rooted post-Pasteur medicine.

If there is one medical scandal emblematic of our time, it is that of Aids, as much for the media hype of which the syndrome is the object as for the dramatic consequences of the faulty interpretation of the immune deficiency phenomena.

Since the appearance in 1981 of what was soon afterwards called "Acquired Immune Deficiency Syndrome" (AIDS), scientists have had all the elements at hand, since the reasons for the weakening of the immune system were fairly well known and explained all the pathologies found: intoxication by illegal chemical or medicinal substances, repeated blood transfusions, malnutrition, prolonged and intense stress….

Against all expectations, these immune deficiency phenomena were attributed to the underhand and damaging action of a previously unknown virus. A virus which even today nobody, among the thousands of researchers who are working non-stop to destroy it, has ever been able to isolate directly from an Aids victim!

Yes! Maybe that seems impossible, extravagant, crazy.

However, despite the rigorous scientific criteria and numerous "official" investigations, nobody has ever been able to establish the least proof that a virus is the cause of AIDS.

Instead of encouraging reasonable experimental verifications, every result from studies that contradict the official hypothesis, either generates new and illogical theories which reinforce the preceding doctrine, or else is rejected outright, or is simply ignored.

Those of you who have been conditioned to believe that AIDS is a sexually transmissible contagious illness, should prepare yourselves for a considerable shock when you read the following chapters and discover the ten lies of Aids.

INTRODUCTION

We have done our utmost to present this work in an easily understandable manner for a non-specialized readership; nevertheless, all claims contained in this book are supported by scientific studies published in journals of high reputation, cited under references at the end.

ETIENNE DE HARVEN, JEAN-CLAUDE ROUSSEZ

LIE #1
AIDS IS A NEW ILLNESS

The public at large as well as the majority of health professionals believe that the AIDS epidemic is a phenomenon which appeared suddenly at the beginning of the 80s, caused by the emergence of a new and terrifying virus.

However, we must remember that from 1981 (the first notification of the syndrome) until 1984 (the announcement of the "discovery" of the virus "responsible" for AIDS), scientists confronted with these sudden collapses of the immune system suspected several reasons for this new pathology, reasons linked to the use of toxic substances and to the life-style of most patients.

Actually, in the United States as well as Western Europe, it was in the male homosexual community that the first cases of non-conventionally acquired immunodeficiency were seen, shortly followed by drug addicts using so-called "hard" IV drugs.

All the symptoms detected in the patients, as well as the pathologies from which they suffered, were obvious consequences of the abuse of narcotics, predominantly nitrites and heroin.

TEN LIES ABOUT AIDS

- **WHAT IS AIDS?**

Acquired immune deficiency syndrome, or AIDS, is not actually one single disease. It is a syndrome, i.e. a collection of signs and symptoms found at the same time in the same patient; in the case of secondary (or acquired) immunodeficiency it is characterized by a severe weakening, or collapse, of the immune defenses. The affected individual becomes, therefore, unable to fight the infections by either endogenous or exogenous germs which are attacking him, and becomes a fragile victim of these opportunistic microbes, as he is incapable of eliminating them.

- **A WELL-KNOWN PHENOMENON**

Acquired immunodeficiency is nothing new, contrary to what the medical establishment would like us to believe. It is a phenomenon that has been known for many years, but which has only been able to be analyzed thanks to new techniques for counting certain families of white cells (CD4- T lymphocytes), cells that are primarily concerned with immune defenses.

For a long time, the two main causes of acquired immunodeficiency were strongly suspected:

- malnutrition
- the use of certain substances harmful to the immune system (drugs, certain medicines, blood transfusions)

We will see later that these two factors are quite sufficient to explain the majority of known cases of AIDS throughout the world.

For the sake of thoroughness, it must be added that immunodeficiency can also be caused by intense and prolonged stress, by certain cancers affecting the lymphatic system, as well as by exposure to electro-magnetic radiation (treatment by cobalt therapy, for example).

Since time immemorial, periods of food shortages and famine have been responsible for widespread death amongst populations.

AIDS IS A NEW ILLNESS

"They died of hunger!" we said, and that was the literal truth. Nevertheless, a good number among them were overwhelmed by multiple and varied opportunistic infections caused by their immunodeficiency. But in those old days, no methodology was available to scientifically measure immune defenses.

As for substances harmful for the immune system, the spread of drug addiction went hand in hand with the progress of medicine.

The first relatively recent cases of acquired immunodeficiency appeared as a side-effect of organ transplant techniques.

In effect, when an organ is transplanted into an individual, it is regarded as a foreign body by his immune system, which tries to eliminate it (that is its purpose).

In order to avoid rejection of the transplant, chemical substances which are designed to seriously weaken their immunity are given to the patients.

These medicines are called "immunosuppressive drugs".

The collapse of the immune system which follows their use is therefore deliberately caused, in the hope of keeping the transplanted patient alive.

It is from there that the first cases of modern acquired immunodeficiency came, years before the official appearance of the "AIDS" syndrome.

Other classes of medicines are equally capable of causing immunodeficiency.

Antibiotics, for example, when abused in the long term, damage the lymphocytes, a family of white blood cells.

As for corticoids, they cause these lymphocytes to leak out of the circulating blood and hide in the tissues. This results in a lowering of the efficiency of the immune system, due to the fact that these cells are not found where they are needed.

Narcotics are by far the main cause of immunodeficiency found in developed countries.

Heavy drug-users have a double reason to be immuno-depressed. On the one hand, the substances that they inject (heroin) or inhale (crack) are cell poisons. In addition, drug addicts are very frequently suffering from malnutrition.

But there is another type of drug abuse linked to the lifestyle of certain homosexual communities, primarily in the United States.

Sexual liberation at the end of the 70s brought about a real explosion at the heart of the gay galaxy. Fear of discrimination and misunderstanding was replaced by a diametrically opposed attitude: the well-known "gay pride".

This wind of freedom was the engine which drove a new and totally uninhibited lifestyle, above all in cities like New York, San Francisco or Los Angeles.

All types of drugs circulated openly in the gay meeting places (bar backrooms, nightclubs, saunas) and beyond. The most prized amongst them were "poppers", inhaled nitrites which are devastating to the immune system and blood vessels.

The ravages caused by all these substances, and their implication in AIDS, will be analyzed in detail in the following chapters.

- **THE LYMPHOCYTE KILLER**

When the first cases of AIDS were analyzed, a common characteristic was found in all the patients: a serious reduction of the T-CD4+ lymphocytes (or, more simply, T4) in the circulating blood (the technique for counting these cells had been developed a short time earlier).

The same condition, however, was later found in numerous seropositive people who had not developed AIDS. Still, the surprising explanation of the phenomenon was that this reduction of T4 cells was characteristic of the action of a virus which targeted this category of immune cells. Thus a reduction in T4 became an indicator of the progress of the infection. In the early 1990s, the number of 200 cells per cubic millimeter of blood became officially part of the diagnostic evidence for any AIDS case in the US and the rest of the world (but not in Canada).

However, there is a persisting mystery, because nobody has ever been able to show that this depletion of T4 could be due to a virus. On the contrary, cell cultures supposedly infected by "HIV", the so-called human immunodeficiency virus, show no loss of the T4 cells that they contain. And, no retrovirus, in the

AIDS IS A NEW ILLNESS

memory of any virologist, had ever caused the death of a host-cell. "HIV" was therefore presented as a very different case.

In fact, it is because certain lymphocytes have a very long life expectancy that it was claimed that they were the target of "HIV". Otherwise, the official theory would not have held up, the other blood cells having too short a life expectancy to explain the virus remaining hidden and inactive for years.

As a matter of fact, low levels of T4 can be associated with a number of conditions such as infections, malnutrition, blood disorders, tuberculosis, stress, pregnancy, the use of corticosteroids.... For example, almost a third of people suffering from severe pneumonia are shown to have a T4 count of less than 200 per cubic millimeter.

There are also perfectly fit people, in good health, who permanently have a low level of T4, for no apparent reason.

Besides, the theory of the virus "killer of T4" was questioned a long time ago, when Luc Montagnier (the discoverer of "HIV") said, at the 68th conference of the University of All Knowledge, Paris, on 8th March 2000[1*]:

> *"In the beginning, we naïvely believed that the cells infected by the virus were dead. In vitro observations using viral strains isolated from patients with confirmed AIDS were leading in that direction. On the other hand, viruses isolated at the early and silent stage of the illness do not kill T4 lymphocytes. The death of the cells is therefore not necessarily directly linked to the infection and to the viral multiplication which exhausts the host-cell. Some indirect mechanisms must be implicated in the cell death."*

Moreover, this quote twice mentions "isolated viruses", which is an abuse of scientific language, because no researcher has ever directly isolated particles of "HIV".

Continuing his explanation of how the virus is supposed to

---

1 * This conférence, held in French, was recorded. It can be watched in streaming video on the website of CANAL-U, at the following address :
http://www.canal-u.fr/canalu/chainev2/utls/programme/68/sequence_id/989273/format_id/3003/

destroy the immune system, Luc Montagnier enumerated those indirect mechanisms which could be held responsible for the reduction in the T4 count: cytotoxic cells of the immune system which destroy the infected cells or those which have fixed the proteins of the viral envelope to their surface; apoptosis (programmed cell suicide).

He finished his presentation with a revealing concession:

> *"We can see that the mechanisms of the illness are highly complex and far from being completely understood."*

In fact, the so-called virus does so little damage to T4 cells that even in a patient in the terminal phase, one can detect its presence in only one cell in a thousand or ten thousand, which is evidently insignificant and most unlikely to cause immune deficiency.

LIE # 2
THERE IS AN AIDS VIRUS: HIV

When searching for the truth, the best method of investigation is without doubt that used in police enquiries, because it has been proved to work. The main criteria to take into account are the following:

- don't be fooled by appearances which are often misleading
- don't trust testimonies from people involved in the matter at hand, either closely or distantly, above all if they could have a motive, or are prone to making subjective judgments
- see who profits from the crime
- check the alibis of the people concerned
- and above all, verify the facts, point by point

If we use this method in seeking the criminal called "HIV", or human immunodeficiency virus, supposedly responsible of AIDS, we will have one surprise after another.

Here is our line of enquiry.

APPEARANCES ARE DECEPTIVE

Have the countless researchers who work all over the world on the AIDS virus, or the thousands of scientific articles published on the subject, managed to prove the existence of the aforesaid virus?

The answer is: no!

In fact, when we take the time (and much is needed) to read the scientific literature relative to the virus itself, we are struck to find that none of these investigations has ever managed to produce direct evidence of the presence of any retroviral particle in an AIDS patient.

However, the techniques are simple and classic, and were perfected well before the advent of molecular biology and genetics. They consist of either direct isolation from the patients, or the infection of laboratory-cultivated cells which are susceptible to infection by a particular virus, like monkey's kidney cells in the case of the poliovirus.

The concentration of the viruses by high-speed centrifugation, the elimination of bacteria and cell debris by ultra-filtration, and the direct observation of the viral particles with an electron microscope are the basis of all classic virology and have been crucial in the confirmation of the viral origin of numerous illnesses.

Seen with an electron microscope, all viruses do not look alike. Their different families (smallpox, herpes, flu, polio, etc.) all have their own morphology. Moreover the classification of the different families of virus is based primarily on the morphology of the viral particles as seen with the electron microscope, relying on observations made in the 1950s to the 1960s. On the other hand, within one given viral family all the particles show remarkably stable dimensions and morphologies which leave no room for doubt or for any confusion. Seen through an electron microscope, there is no possibility that particles of herpes virus could be confused with smallpox, for example.

So, when one succeeds in concentrating a given virus with a very great degree of purity, and when this "purified" virus is observed with an electron microscope, the first thing that

THERE IS AN AIDS VIRUS: HIV

strikes the viewer is the extreme homogeneity of this population of particles which all have almost exactly the same diameter and the same structure or morphology.

It isn't always easy to purify a given virus to a very high degree, mainly because it isn't always simple to eliminate contamination of the preparations by cell debris.

However, when successful viral purification is indisputably confirmed by electron microscopy, it is then possible to entrust these samples to biochemists, who can then isolate molecules (proteins, enzymes, nucleic acids) whose actual viral origin is guaranteed by the purity of the initial sample. Such molecules could then, *and only then*, be considered as specific "molecular markers". In those cases, but only in those cases, the rigorous identification of a viral "molecular marker" becomes equivalent to the identification of the virus itself.

Such rational research steps produced, in the 50s-60s, famous examples in the study of viral particles associated with certain leukemias, and certain cancers in several types of laboratory animals, mainly mice and chickens. They mostly concerned RNA viruses, later named "retroviruses", a viral family to which the hypothetical "HIV" belongs.

As a matter of fact, from the blood of chickens and mice suffering from leukemia, it became possible to isolate and purify innumerable viral particles that have all more or less the same diameter (110 nanometers), and were capable of transmitting leukemia to healthy animals.

This success had an immense impact on establishing priorities in cancer research during the 60s and 70s.

How could it be that these viruses, so readily isolated and purified in mice and chickens, could never be found in human leukemias?

Of mice and men ....

Such viruses have **never** been identified in any human illness, as infectious agents capable of transmitting the same disease to laboratory animals. In spite of the fact that research programs in this direction, mainly in the United States, received massive grant support (the "war against cancer" of Richard Nixon,

1972), it all led to nothing, and this failure began to be glaringly obvious in 1980-81.

This was just at the time of the emergence of AIDS.

Was this new pathology offering an ultimate chance for research on human "retroviruses"? In this expectation, numerous fundamental cancerology laboratories in the United States and in Europe suddenly began to concentrate their research on AIDS, supported by massive increases in research grants. As a consequence, the hypothesis of the isolation of a retrovirus as the "probable" cause of AIDS was precipitously formulated in 1983-1984. The AIDS virus had been "invented" (as characterized by Peter Duesberg in his 1996 book).

This was politically correct but scientifically absurd.

Scientific integrity took a back seat in this adventure. Pressure groups, the media and the pharmaceutical giants quickly saw the huge potential profit to be made from this pseudo-scientific development, in what will probably remain the blackest page in the history of medicine.

Because "HIV" remains a radically unproven hypothesis. If it wasn't for the formidable media hype suggesting its causality in the pathology of AIDS, no credibility would have been given to the existence of this microbe which was, and still is, hypothetical. Our enquiry shall further consolidate this analysis.

THE "DISCOVERY" OF THE VIRUS

It was a team from the Pasteur Institute, led by Professor Luc Montagnier which was the first to announce, in 1983, the discovery of a retrovirus from samples taken from a "pre-AIDS" patient.

The following year, Robert Gallo in the United States made a similar announcement. Later it was shown that Gallo had misrepresented as "his discovery" a cell culture sample which Luc Montagnier had generously given him several months before. The same mishap happened to Robin Weiss, the well known British AIDS specialist, who was obliged to acknowledge that his own discovery of the virus resulted from the fact that he, too, had received a culture sample from Luc Montagnier.

THERE IS AN AIDS VIRUS: HIV

It is noticeable that, on both sides of the Atlantic the three topmost teams on the subject, after more than two years of research had only been able to announce a vague presumption as a result of studying cell cultures that all had originated from one single patient!

Presumption, because if one keeps to the established facts, these teams have never announced that they isolated a new virus shown to be the cause of AIDS. Neither, anywhere in all the medical literature, is there a single article to be found, showing a conclusion that such a retrovirus has been isolated, and that this virus *is* the cause of AIDS.

REVERSE TRANSCRIPTASE

In 1970, Howard Temin and David Baltimore announced (independently and simultaneously) the discovery of a new enzyme: *reverse transcriptase*. They would later win the Nobel Prize for medicine in 1975 for their discovery on this enzyme.

Just for the record, its real discoverer was probably the French researcher Mirko Beljanski, a brilliant French biologist, who was very badly rewarded for his original research contributions.

In what way was this new enzyme revolutionary?

Cell nuclei contain all their genetic information encoded in long double-stranded molecules of DNA (deoxyribonucleic acid). In order to manufacture a particular type of protein, DNA creates a copy of its numerous sequences, by means of an enzyme called RNA polymerase. This chemically distinct copy, destined to effect the transmission of the genetic message, is made of RNA (ribonucleic acid).

Initial dogma held that only the transcription of DNA into RNA was possible, thanks to the action of RNA polymerase. And yet in 1970 the breakthrough was that reverse transcriptase activity demonstrated possible synthesis of DNA from an RNA template, thereby falsifying the one-way hypothesis dogmatically imposed until then.

The enzyme which made this phenomenon possible was logically baptized "reverse transcriptase". Without waiting for the results of numerous control experiments which this revolutionary observation called for, the activity of this enzyme observed supposedly in purified samples of the virus associated with certain leukemias and cancers in mice and chickens (see above) was presented as a specific molecular marker of these viruses.

This family of virus was, therefore, re-baptized "retrovirus".

The problem was that neither Temin nor Baltimore had verified the purity of the virus samples in which they had identified the enzymatic activity in question. Yet a short while after their publications in 1970, it became evident that reverse transcription was a widespread phenomenon in biology. From 1971 it was apparent that reverse transcription was common to a great number of animal cells, as well as bacteria (Beljanski).

Consequently, before considering the enzyme as a "retroviral marker", the experiments of Temin and Baltimore needed to be repeated on samples whose degree of purification would have been verified, in order to exclude the presence of cell debris that could, by themselves, explain the observed reverse transcriptase activity.

These controls were never carried out, and consequently for more than thirty years the reverse transcriptase (RT) enzyme has been erroneously considered the principal molecular marker of retroviruses.

THE 1.16 BAND

Two methods have been successfully used to purify viruses, that is to say to isolate them from anything else. One is based on ultra-filtration, the other on ultra-centrifugation.

The first method consists of filtering a preparation through special filters, blocking particles above a certain dimension.

The ancestor of these selective filters used to isolate very small microbes (for this reason known at the time as "virus filtrants") is that invented at the end of the 19th century by Charles Chamberland, a colleague of Louis Pasteur.

The second method uses high speed centrifugation. Progressively, and as this operation is carried out, the preparation separates into different layers ("bands") according to the density of the elements which it comprises. In the same way that the density of pure water is 1 gram per milliliter (or 1 kilogram per liter), the density band at which retroviruses sediment in a solution of sucrose is 1.16 g/ml.

The problem with the method of density gradients, abundantly used by research laboratories, is that retroviruses are not the only particulate elements that sediment in this band of 1.16 g/ml. Cell debris, such as "microvesicles", sediment at the same level in the same gradient.

Therefore collecting material at this density is not sufficient to proclaim the isolation of a retrovirus, far from it!

It is therefore absolutely essential to ascertain the absence of cell debris by electron microscopy, a fact that was clearly highlighted in 1973, at the Pasteur Institute, during a major conference dealing exclusively with the methods of purifying retroviruses (study published in the *Spectra 2000* review, No. 4, pages 237 to 243, under the title *"Purification and partial differentiation of the particles of murine sarcoma virus (M. MSV) according to their sedimentation rates in sucrose density gradient"*).

ISOLATION OF THE VIRUS

In the historic article published in 1983 by Françoise Barré-Sinoussi, Jean-Claude Chermann, Luc Montagnier and their colleagues *"Isolation of a T-lymphotropic retrovirus from a patient at risk for acquired immune deficiency syndrome [AIDS]" – Science*, volume 220 of 20th May 1983, pages 868 to 871, in which the isolation of a retrovirus was announced, the detection of the enzymatic activity of reverse transcriptase in a fraction sedimenting at 1.16 g/ml was the key data used to demonstrate that a retrovirus was indeed present. Yet we know now that this enzyme is not a specific marker of retroviruses! And we have known for a very long time that the fractions 1.16 g/ml contain an abundance of cell debris, perfectly capable of explaining the presence of the enzymatic activity ......

This article also made a big case out of an electron micrograph illustrating retroviruses growing on the surface of a lymphocyte. The image was interpreted as proof of the infection of the cultured cells by some material that had been obtained from the patient.

What the article omitted to consider is that the cultures were mixed with lymphocytes taken from umbilical cord blood, and that the human placenta has been known for several years as a tissue exceptionally rich in endogenous human retroviruses (manufactured by the cells), or HERVs.

In short, this article considered all over the world as the classic, historical reference on the isolation of "HIV" is based on three basic methodological mistakes:

1 - Not having verified by electron microscopy the absence of cell debris in the analyzed samples;

2 – Having ignored the possible enzymatic activity of cell debris;

3 - Having ignored the highly probable contribution of endogenous retroviruses from the placental cells which had been added to the cultures.

This study must therefore be considered as a demonstration (primarily by electron microscopy) of the presence of a retrovirus, probably of endogenous (placenta) origin, in the analyzed cell cultures. It cannot be regarded, however, as a proof of the isolation of a retrovirus originating from an AIDS patient, and therefore had no reason whatsoever to be even hypothetically linked to the disease.

Most surprisingly, it took fifteen years for the most obvious experimental control experiments to be carried out, in two laboratories, one in the United States and the other in France. These two laboratories jointly published, in *Virology*, the results of their electron microscopic studies of the sucrose gradients obtained from the cell cultures supposed to produce "HIV". In both cases, the authors observed an abundance of cell debris, without any acceptable evidence of retroviral particles. These so-called "purified" viruses really did not deserve to be thus qualified!

At about the same time, Luc Montagnier was interviewed by journalist Djamel Tahi and finally admitted on videotape that

THERE IS AN AIDS VIRUS: HIV

in effect, "HIV" had never been purified in his laboratory.

It is interesting to note that in the article originating from the Pasteur Institute in 1973 and previously cited in reference, there was a clear indication that reverse transcriptase activity was present in cell debris. As astonishing as it may seem, it was in that same Pasteur Institute laboratory that, ten years later, in 1983, the possible enzyme contribution from cell debris was ignored, putting AIDS research onto the wrong track for more than 20 years.

VIRUS "MARKERS"

Outside of the enzymatic activity of reverse transcriptase, which as we have just seen constituted the first (false) sign of the presence of a retrovirus in the cultures taken from an AIDS patient, the presence of certain molecular markers, in this case proteins, was attributed to retroviral activity. There were a dozen of these proteins that were considered peculiar to the so-called "HIV".

We will discuss these proteins again in the chapter about the tests for HIV-positivity, but we can already indicate that their viral origin has never been demonstrated, that on the contrary their specificity has never been verified and that these proteins are normal cell components that should always be expected in contaminating cell debris.

VIRUS "PICTURES"

Journals and magazines all over the world contain admirable pictures, computer-enhanced and in totally artificial colors, supposedly representing "HIV" itself.

Publishing these images is meant to give the public at large, and doctors as well (!), an apparently clear and indisputable message: "HIV" has effectively been isolated, because we can see it and display it with an electron microscope!

This is an enormous lie!

All these images derive from electron microscopy of cell cultures. None come directly from one single AIDS patient, even if the chosen patients had been labeled as showing a heightened viral load.

Luc Montagnier himself has described the very complex cell cultures used for "HIV" as real "retrovirus soups". How true that is!

On the one hand, everything was set up so that the retroviral particles would appear in these cultures, and on the other hand elementary controls which should have been done to understand the real origin of these viruses were never performed or, if they were, were never the subject of any publication!

It is known that the cell cultures used at the Pasteur Institute in 1983 were always mixed and hyper-stimulated cultures. Mixed, because they were composed of a skilful blend of several cell lines comprising, for example, the patient's lymphocytes, plus the so-called "immortal" cancerous cells, plus lymphocytes from the patient mixed with umbilical cord lymphocytes which, deriving from the placenta, have every likelihood of being carriers of endogenous retroviruses.

An example of how a good electron micrograph is fraudulently used as a convincing force is shown by the previously mentioned classic article of 1983. Indeed, one sees there an excellent image showing particles of retrovirus "budding" on the surface of a lymphocyte.

Perfect! But the authors use this image to prove that this lymphocyte has been infected by the patient's viruses. Yet there is not the faintest proof of that interpretation!

On the contrary, far more likely is the probability that endogenous retroviruses from these placental lymphocytes coming from umbilical cord blood have been activated by the particular conditions of the culture.

All these mixed cultures are excessively hyper-stimulated by different growth factors like phytohemagglutinin (PHA), the growth factor of T lymphocytes (TCGF), as well as interleukin-2, or corticosteroids. Yet all these factors are known as activators of the expression of endogenous retroviruses that we all carry in ourselves, especially in embryonic cells like the placenta.

It is not surprising therefore to observe retroviruses in these hyper-stimulated "retroviral soups".

THERE IS AN AIDS VIRUS: HIV

A NON-RESPECTED PROTOCOL

Ideally, to demonstrate the presence of pathogenic retroviruses in patients, and reflecting the guidelines of Koch's postulates, the following protocol should be applied:

1. From tissue or blood from the patient, virus particles must be isolated and the virus purified, by removing all non-retroviral elements.
2. Verify the purity of the viral sample by electron microscopy, ultra-filtration and centrifugation, and identify the nature of its nucleic acid and proteins.
3. Infect with the purified virus either a susceptible laboratory animal or a cell culture to produce a new generation of virus.
4. Isolate the viral particles from that new generation and demonstrate that they have the same morphological and biochemical characteristics.
5. Verify that the viruses of this new generation have the same pathogenic properties either in susceptible laboratory animal or in an appropriate cell culture.

Admittedly, many well-known human viral diseases would fail to satisfy some of these steps. Unfortunately, however, and as far as HIV research is concerned, the initial key step of isolation and purification has never been satisfactorily demonstrated, making it impossible to follow the above outlined protocol.

VIRUS, WHERE ARE YOU?

We must therefore surrender to the evidence: the alleged "HIV" has never been neither isolated nor purified.

Retroviral particles, most likely of endogenous origin, have been observed in cell cultures, but their hypothetical link with AIDS patients has never been proven any more than their pathogenic potential.

TEN LIES ABOUT AIDS

For political, and not for scientific reasons, the AIDS orthodoxy has tried to deal with this difficulty by forgetting about isolating viral particles and relying instead on hypothetical molecular "markers".

It was vital to save the HIV=AIDS hypothesis, even at the cost of scientific integrity! However, as we shall see later, these markers lack specificity and did not lead to any coherent observations.

If AIDS was effectively an illness caused by a retrovirus, how is it possible that more than twenty years of research have not permitted the isolation of the responsible retrovirus in a scientifically acceptable fashion?

How is it that these same retroviruses that are so easily isolated in leukemic or cancerous mice should be so difficult to find in man?

Dr Kary Mullis (biochemist, Nobel Prize for Chemistry 1993) tried a number of times to obtain from his colleagues references to at least one study that would have shown that "HIV" was the cause of AIDS. This hypothesis being universally accepted, he initially thought that proofs of the causal relationship between HIV and AIDS shouldn't be difficult to find. He was in for a bitter disappointment.

Here is how he described:

> "I did computer searches, but came up with nothing. Of course, you can miss something important in computer searches by not putting in just the right key words. To be certain about a scientific issue, it's best to ask other scientists directly. That's one thing that scientific conferences in faraway places with nice beaches are for.
>
> I was going to a lot of meetings and conferences as part of my job. I got in the habit of approaching anyone who gave a talk about AIDS and asking him or her what reference I should quote for that increasingly problematic statement, "HIV is the probable cause of AIDS."
>
> After ten or fifteen meetings over a couple years, I was getting pretty upset when no one could cite the reference. I didn't like the ugly conclusion that was forming in my mind: The entire campaign against a disease increasingly regarded as a twen-

THERE IS AN AIDS VIRUS: HIV

tieth century Black Plague was based on a hypothesis whose origins no one could recall. That defied both scientific and common sense.

Finally, I had an opportunity to question one of the giants in HIV and AIDS research, Dr Luc Montagnier of the Pasteur Institute, when he gave a talk in San Diego. It would be the last time I would be able to ask my little question without showing anger, and I figured Montagnier would know the answer. So I asked him.

With a look of condescending puzzlement, Montagnier said, "Why don't you quote the report from the Centers for Disease Control?"

I replied, "It doesn't really address the issue of whether or not HIV is the probable cause of AIDS, does it?"

"No," he admitted, no doubt wondering when I would just go away. He looked for support to the little circle of people around him, but they were all awaiting a more definitive response, like I was.

"Why don't you quote the work on SIV [Simian Immunodeficiency Virus]?" the good doctor offered.

"I read that too, Dr Montagnier," I responded. "What happened to those monkeys didn't remind me of AIDS. Besides, that paper was just published only a couple of months ago. I'm looking for the original paper where somebody showed that HIV caused AIDS.

This time, Dr Montagnier's response was to walk quickly away to greet an acquaintance across the room ".

Let us point out, as an anecdote, the following fact which nicely demonstrates how fiercely official research wants to save the viral theory of AIDS: in June 2000, a researcher published in the prestigious journal *Science* an article in which he announced that analysis of the "molecular clock" of "HIV" had allowed him to trace the birth date of the virus (or very nearly) to 1931, the event having taken place in Africa (evidently!).

It would be interesting to ask him two questions:

- How had he managed to decipher the molecular clock of a virus that nobody had ever been able to isolate?

- Would he be capable, by analyzing the clock of his own cells, to find the date on which his own AIDS (Acquired Intelligence-Deficiency Syndrome) had begun?

A JOURNEY TO THE LAND OF MUTANTS!

For more than two decades, researchers have been trying to decipher the genome of the alleged "HIV". In vain! Despite the state-of-the-art technological arsenal available to them, they are incapable of drawing up its genetic card.

First of all, nobody is in agreement with anybody else on the number of genes that are contained in the genome of the virus. Some say that there are eight; others say nine; still others estimate them at ten.

Also, attempts to decode the genome's sequences produce such disparate elements that no two laboratories in the world can produce similar results.

According to a study published in 1996, the differences could amount to 40% of the genome!

In order to emphasize the enormity of these differences, one should point out that among the human races in all their diversity, the genome does not vary by more than one in a thousand. The genomic variation between a man and a primate is no more than 2%. Between a man and an elephant, this difference is around 30%.

Let us state this loud and clear: nobody has ever found two identical HIV viral genomes in the same patient!

From that to believing that the genomes in question are not those of a virus but come from different and varied cell debris, there is just one step ... that the tens of thousands of scientists living from the AIDS-business are careful to keep to themselves.

The viral AIDS lobby has decided otherwise, and chooses to explain these colossal differences by the fact that the virus hasn't finished mutating.

However, virologists well know that when a virus mutates, the mutation only differs from the original in a negligible proportion.

THERE IS AN AIDS VIRUS: HIV

Never mind! They have accepted this nonsense hook, line and sinker.

And since one can probably exaggerate here without much fear of contradiction, we should not hesitate to mention some figures which defy all logic: according to researchers at the Pasteur Institute, an HIV-positive asymptomatic patient can harbour at least a million genetically distinct variants of "HIV". In a confirmed AIDS patient, this figure can reach a hundred million variants!

Wake up Hippocrates, they've gone mad!

LIE #3
HIV IS THE CAUSE OF AIDS

Despite the colossal budget spent in the fight against AIDS and an unprecedented mobilization of the research world, the syndrome continues its ravages, killing a huge number of individuals every year. Why this failure?

The answer is two-fold. Firstly, the dogmatic acceptance of the viral hypothesis has totally eclipsed the real causes of AIDS. Secondly, the medicinal treatments prescribed to patients as well as to asymptomatic HIV-positives individuals are dangerously toxic, as we shall see in the following chapter.

The first cases of AIDS observed in the early 1980s in the United States were all detected within the homosexual community and intravenous drug users. The health authorities, like the health professionals, should have suspected that they were facing immune collapses caused by the absorption of drugs, since drug abuse was common to all the patients.

This sensible interpretation was seriously considered until 1984, the date of the announcement of the discovery of an infectious agent, "HIV" (the human deficiency virus, then called "HTLV III"), to which exclusive responsibility for the syndrome was attributed.

It was only then that the public at large was warned of a new and terrible plague that was threatening mankind, and thanks to very well-orchestrated media hype the result was to cause a feeling of terror in the general population and a wind of panic in the homosexual community.

As Coluche once said: "AIDS is transmitted by the media." Once again, the great French comedian had got it right!

MULTIPLE CAUSES

There are currently about thirty illnesses listed as being AIDS-defining, several of which have nothing to do with immunodeficiency.

These illnesses don't strike randomly, but are strongly linked to a particular type of patient. For example, Kaposi's sarcoma only affects homosexuals addicted to certain drugs, above all nitrites; pneumocytosis is found essentially in intravenous drug users and crack smokers; hemophiliacs are primarily vulnerable to pneumonia and fungal infections.

It is clear that each group of "at risk" individuals develops the pathologies typical for that group. If a virus were the cause of AIDS, it would provoke these illnesses in a totally random distribution.

The same would be expected in the geographical epidemiology of AIDS-linked infections. However, the illnesses found in Western countries don't match those found in developing countries.

IN HOMOSEXUALS

The fact of being homosexual is not by itself an AIDS risk factor. It is only the life-style of certain male homosexuals that can cause immunodeficiency.

After homosexuality was decriminalized in the USA, the decade of the 70s was an euphoric period during which liberated homosexuals closed ranks and began to establish their own communities, even creating their own villages in the heart of the big cities. This life-style pattern subsequently developed in Western Europe.

Gay meeting places multiplied and nightlife intensified, leading to numerous encounters that resulted in sexual relations as frequent as they were transitory.

Different drugs circulated freely (cannabis, cocaine, amphetamines, LSD, barbiturates, heroin...), but the undisputed stars were "poppers", small ampoules of amyl nitrite, a powerful vasodilator apparently possessing aphrodisiac properties.

Originally, amyl nitrite was used as an arterial dilator in the treatment of coronary diseases. From the 60s, the homosexual community diverted nitrites from their medicinal use and nitrite addiction became extremely popular. Affordably priced, the principal advantage of poppers was to relax the anal sphincter, reducing pain caused by repetitive penetration, maintaining erection and intensifying orgasm, all effects of particular interest for fast-track homosexuals.

The effect of nitrites being short-lived, they had to be inhaled frequently.

To get an idea of the atmosphere at the time in homosexual communities in the big cities, this is what John Lauristen, a well-known gay activist and scholar, had to say when he was interviewed by dissident journalist Liam Scheff (extract):

> "I lived in New York from '63 to '95; I was there, right in the heart of it. I lived around the corner from an extremely popular gay club called The Saint. On some nights, a couple thousand men would show up. The main activity was consuming drugs of every sort: ecstasy, poppers, marijuana, quaaludes, MDA, crystal meth, LSD, cocaine and designer drugs. Some drugs only showed up once, like the one they made specially for the club's opening night.
>
> At clubs like The Saint, there was a drug schedule. Someone would say, "Now it's time for ecstasy, now it's time for crystal, now it's time for Special K," and hundreds to a couple thousand guys would all do drugs at the same time. This went on all evening. They mixed this with alcohol through the course of the long, long night. A drug called "poppers" was used constantly, because it was cheap and legal.
>
> ... They were used ubiquitously. They came in little vials that you'd pop open and snort. Some gay men used poppers first thing in the morning, on the dance floor and every time they had sex. At gay discotheques, men shuffled around in a daze, holding their poppers bottles under their nose. The acrid odour of poppers was synonymous with gay gathering places".

Nitrites, the active agents of poppers, are dangerous poisons which cause, amongst other things damage to the lungs and heart, fungal infections, neurological disorders, genetic mutations, and above all immune deficiencies, by their action on the bone marrow where blood cells are manufactured.

Once they are in the blood, nitrites convert themselves into nitric oxide and damage the internal walls of the blood vessels, which explain their implication in cancer of the capillaries such as Kaposi's sarcoma.

Although now illegal, poppers are still available today, whether under innocent pseudonyms such as "leather cleaner", or sold openly, for example in sex shops.

Nitrite addiction became an even more serious problem when poppers began to be used by heterosexuals seeking increased sexual performance.

Despite evidence that the use of poppers was associated with the majority of AIDS cases among homosexuals, in the United States, since 1983 public health organizations pressurized certain media within the gay community into totally absolving nitrites. This attitude could be regarded as criminal.

It wasn't until 1994 that Robert Gallo, "co-discoverer" of "HIV" and promoter of the first antibody screening test, admitted during a NIDA conference (*National Institute on Drug Abuse*) that Kaposi's sarcoma, a typical illness among the homosexual community, was probably not caused by a virus, but that poppers were likely the main culprit.

This belated confession did nothing to change official policies.

However, the implication of nitrites in the occurrence of Kaposi's sarcoma had been shown on numerous occasions. As Dr Peter Duesberg recalled in a lengthy article which appeared in 1992 in the journal *Pharmacology and Therapeutics*, the lowering of nitrite consumption correlates with a lower incidence of Kaposi's sarcoma amongst AIDS patients.

For example, poppers were taken by 58% of homosexuals in San Francisco in 1984, against 27% in 1991. Similarly, the incidence of Kaposi's sarcoma in AIDS patients, which was 50% in 1981 (the first year of AIDS), fell to 37% in 1983, and was less than 10% in 1991.

This lowering in the consumption of inhaled nitrites is ex-

HIV IS THE CAUSE OF AIDS

plained by the fact that despite the officially circulated information, there was awareness within the homosexual community that the toxicity of poppers had a prejudicial effect on health.

The intensive use of various drugs was (and still is) the principal factor in immunodeficiency among male homosexuals. The best documented article on the subject was published in June 2003 in the *Journal of Biosciences*, authored by Duesberg, Rasnick and Koehnlein. This article, entitled *"The chemical causes of AIDS"*, cited an official study from the CDC (*Centers for Disease Control and Prevention*, an organization responsible for the surveillance of infectious illnesses in the United States) produced in 1983 (thus at the beginning of AIDS), regarding the use of drugs by homosexuals in the United States. Table 1 shows part of the results of this inquiry, giving the frequencies of consumption of various drugs in a group of 170 male homosexual, of whom 50 already suffered from AIDS.

Drugs taken	Percentage of users
Inhaled nitrites (poppers)	96%
Ethylchloride	35% to 50%
Cocaine	50% to 60%
Amphetamines	50% to 70%
PCP (Phenylcyclidine)	40%
LSD (Lysergic diethylamide acid)	40% to 60%
Methaqualone (psychotropic medication)	40% to 60%
Barbiturates	25%
Marijuana	90%
Heroin	10%
No drugs	No reported cases

Table 1: Use of drugs from a sample of male homosexuals in the United States in 1983.

Another likely cause of immunodeficiency particular to male homosexuals with multiple partners is the excessive use of antibiotics.

Undoubtedly, having sex without a condom, and the culpable negligence of certain carriers of sexually transmissible diseases have propagated infections like syphilis and gonorrhea.

Antibiotics constitute an excellent therapy for these illnesses, but end up, when treatment extends over a long time, causing severe damage to the body. Certain homosexuals, from fear of becoming re-infected, even take these antibiotics as a preventative measure, and end up being under permanent treatment.

While impeding the proliferation of bacteria, antibiotics also interfere with certain functions related to cell replication, which leads in particular to immune deficiency.

Moreover, various studies done since the 1970s have shown that highly promiscuous male homosexuals constituted a group at high risk of contracting numerous infections, in the United States as well as in Europe.

Since 1969, an antibiotic with two components of which the generic name is cotrimoxazol (better known under the brand names of Septrim® and Bactrim®) was seen as the most effective weapon against many infectious diseases. It was therefore used abundantly by the homosexual community as a miracle remedy.

Unfortunately, this antibiotic is a frightening immunosuppresor, as tests carried out a little later in England confirmed.

It was also shown in 1971 that candidiasis, one of the illnesses symptomatic of AIDS, could appear after treatment with cotrimoxazol, even in sero-negative individuals. It was also shown in 1981 that this antibiotic caused serious damage at the level of cellular DNA and mitochondria.

IN DRUG ADDICTS

Using "recreational" drugs (as opposed to medicinal drugs) causes serious health problems in the medium to long term, in particular immunodeficiency and the appearance of ailments defined as being AIDS related, such as tuberculosis, pneumonia, neurological disorders, weight loss, persistent fever, lymphadenopathy...

HIV IS THE CAUSE OF AIDS

This is nothing new, however! As long ago as 1909, a French study produced evidence indicating high susceptibility to infections among drug addicts, at a time when drug addiction was, however, not as widespread as it is now. So, we cannot say today: "We didn't know..."

This study was followed by many others, all equally conclusive, which makes the attitude of the organizations and professionals in charge of public health unforgivable, when they had the likely evidence for the chemical origin of AIDS before their eyes, at least in the case of drug addicts.

Long-term effects of opiates are cumulative, which explains why it takes several years for drug addicts to exhibit these illnesses that are erroneously attributed to a "slow" virus.

The long-term use of psychoactive drugs is therefore sufficient to explain AIDS in serious drug addicts. Unfortunately, such addictions are often accompanied by an important aggravating cofactor that will precipitate a clinical downhill course, which is malnutrition. Malnutrition is indeed a standard phenomenon, almost inevitable in many heroin addicts. Taking narcotics becomes such a dominating obsession that appetite is lost. Yet malnutrition alone, as we will see later, has been recognized for a long time as an important cause of immune deficiency.

IN HEMOPHILIACS

Hemophilia is a hereditary genetic illness in which the blood does not coagulate effectively. In the case of an injury or rupture of a blood vessel, severe bleeding is inevitable.

The coagulation process requires the action of a series of proteins called "coagulation factors". In hemophiliacs, there is a shortage or absence of some of these factors.

Hemophilia is a serious illness that cannot be cured, but which is controlled on a day-to-day basis with perfusions of the missing coagulation factors and, in the case of hemorrhage, by blood transfusions. Although treatment protocols and the quality of transfused products are constantly being improved, severe hemophilia is frequently fatal.

Preventative treatment for hemophiliacs with the aid of

replacement coagulation factors has been in use since 1969. However, facing the intrusion of large amounts of transfused foreign proteins, the immune system reacts by manufacturing antibodies against them. The more antibodies are produced, the more the dose of the coagulation factors has to be increased. This really becomes then a double-edged sword that in the long term leads to exhaustion of the immune system.

Moreover, in the numerous cases where hemophiliacs receive multiple blood transfusions as well, a large increase in the production of antibodies and a severe immune deficiency can frequently be expected.

In addition, the liver, which is in the front line in the elimination of metabolic waste, is the organ most affected by these repeated injections. This explains the death of many hemophiliacs following hepatic failures, especially before the improvement in the purification techniques of products extracted from blood products and the manufacture of coagulation factors stemming from biotechnologies (recombinant factors).

It is therefore absolutely pointless to consider a hypothetical contamination of transfused blood by a hypothetical "HIV" to explain phenomena that were observed years before AIDS.

Finally, as we shall see in the next chapter, the high mortality rate recorded amongst hemophiliacs after 1987 can readily be explained by the fact that, from that year on, many seropositive hemophiliacs were treated with high dosages of AZT, and not because they were the victims of a so-called HIV infection originating from "contaminated" transfused blood.

THE MALNOURISHED

Serious and long-term food deprivation is responsible for the majority of cases of immunodeficiency throughout the world, which readily explains why AIDS in the poor countries (in Africa, particularly) has nothing in common with AIDS in the developed countries.

As we have already stated, it has been known for almost a century that malnutrition is the principal cause of immune deficiency. A sufficient and balanced diet provides the body with essential elements like water, energy-supplying substances (proteins and calories), vitamins and minerals. It is above all a lack of protein that damages the immune system.

In underprivileged populations, food deprivation can start during fetal life, when the future mother, under-nourished herself, cannot supply the necessary substances for the normal growth of the fetus.

Under-nourished people suffer from an atrophy of the lymphoid tissues (the reservoirs of the immune cells) and particularly the thymus, the place of maturation of T lymphocytes, whose size can be considerably reduced in children. The cellular immunity finds itself reduced in proportion to the degree of under-nourishment. In the Intertropical zone, protein deficit is further accentuated by the presence of endemic illnesses that affect the digestive system, in particular diarrhea.

These immune deficiencies are, however, reversible, since adequate feeding (when available...) can re-establish normal lymphocyte functions in a few months.

LIE #4
ANTIVIRAL MEDICATION IS BENEFICIAL

Between 1981 and 1986, the medical authorities applied themselves to treating AIDS patients by fighting, one by one, the infections of which they were victims.

Admittedly, this method was not crowned with success. In effect, in desperate cases the battle was unequal, even useless, and in less severe cases the benefit of the treatments was often undermined by the patients themselves going back to the lifestyle that was destroying their immune system, as soon as they left hospital.

In 1987 the first alleged antiviral medication specifically for the treatment of AIDS became available: AZT. The following year saw the mortality rate of patients rocketing. This very sudden increase in the mortality rate was particularly noticeable in a group of HIV-positive hemophiliacs studied in the United Kingdom (See Darby, 1995, under reference). Rather than seeing a causal relationship between the toxicity of AZT and the disaster, the phenomenon was attributed to an increase of "HIV" virulence.

According to the official hypothesis, the "HIV" retrovirus introduces itself into certain immune cells (CD4 lymphocytes) whose genetic material it uses in order to replicate. The genome of the virus, constituted of RNA, is transcribed into DNA (called proviral DNA) that inserts itself into the cellular genome. The result is the manufacture of innumerable copies of this proviral DNA as well as the associated proteins, later assembled to form new viruses.

The action of several enzymes is necessary in these processes:

- reverse transcriptase, which synthesizes DNA from the RNA;
- integrase, which allows the insertion of proviral DNA in the genome of the cell;
- proteases, which are involved in the assembly of the newly replicated viruses.

Any antiviral medication would therefore have to interfere with one or several of these steps. Unfortunately, all substances capable of inhibiting DNA synthesis equally prevent the synthesis of cellular DNA, which is to say the genome itself, thus blocking cell reproduction, and killing the cells!

By killing lymphatic cells, antiviral medications act as "immunosuppressors", causing or aggravating the immunodeficiency that they are supposed to fight.

AZT

Azidothymidine, or AZT, was first discovered in the early 60s and suggested for cancer chemotherapy. Its devastating effects (systematically lethal in laboratory mice!) met with a categorical rejection by the authorities responsible for the accreditation of new anti-cancer medications.

Other times, other customs: with a most pressing need to provide a therapy for AIDS patients coming as much from the political side as from the medical body and the influential homosexual lobby, a surprising authorization was given to put AZT on the market as a matter of emergency, despite its very high toxicity.

Doses of up to 1.8 grams per day were authorized, which is

ANTIVIRAL MEDICATION IS BENEFICIAL

most surprising in view of the extreme toxicity of this molecule. The most compelling analysis of AZT toxicity has been published in 2000 by Anthony Brink (See "Debating AZT" by Anthony Brink under References).

During transcription of retroviral RNA to DNA, just as in the replication of the cell genome, AZT introduces itself into the new DNA chain during synthesis, blocking its elongation and thus preventing replication.

For this reason AZT (as well as the other members of this pharmaceutical family) is called a DNA chain "terminator".

Not being selective, this operation doesn't only prevent viral replication but also the reproduction of many cells in the body. Consequently, tissues in which cell divisions are extremely frequent, like the digestive tract mucosa and the bone marrow, are drastically affected by AZT. This explains the most alarming number of digestive and hematological side effects observed in patients exposed to this "medication".

OTHER ANTI-VIRALS

AZT is part of the "nucleoside analog reverse transcriptase inhibitors" family. These anti-virals are known under the generic names of ddC (*zalcitabine*), ddI (*didanosine*), d4T (*stavudine*), 3TC (*lamivudine*), *abacavir, ganciclovir, tenofovir* ...

Each has its own molecular action mode, but the principle is always the same. They function as "antimetabolites", i.e. affecting synthesis of nucleic acid molecules.

What are the "undesirable" effects of this family of anti-retrovirals?

- General effects: fatigue, fever, nausea, visual troubles, anxiety, insomnia, depression, loss of appetite, weight loss, muscle and joint pains, aches, skin rashes, alopecia (hair loss), muscular dystrophy, decreased libido;
- Effects on the blood: reduction in the number of red cells, of white cells (immunodepression), lowering of the hemoglobin level, increase in the volume of red corpuscles, bone

marrow alterations (where blood cells are manufactured), increase in triglycerides and cholesterol, lactic acidosis;
- Effects on certain organs: pancreatitis, liver failure, gastro-intestinal troubles (vomiting, diarrhea), respiratory problems, lesions of the head of some bones like the femur (avascular necrosis), esophageal or mouth ulcers;
- Effects on the nervous system: paresthesias (numbness, pain, pins and needles, tingling...), epilepsy, dementia.

These are possible effects but which, happily, are not all found in the same individual, certain of them being, moreover, very rare. Nevertheless, some of these ailments can be very serious, even lethal. They include medullary aplasia (destruction of the bone marrow) and mitochondrial dysfunction (small organelles which constitute the energy power-station of the cells) that causes cellular anoxia and leads to a dangerous excess of lactic acid in the blood.

Moreover, when these medications are administered to a pregnant woman, they may cause abortion, malformations of the fetus, brain damage or other serious health and growth problems of the infant.

The second large antiviral family used in AIDS is called "non-nucleoside analog reverse transcriptase inhibitors", another complicated name signifying that they directly alter this enzyme activity, without presenting a genetic trap for DNA.

The principal drugs belonging to this family are known under the names of *nevirapine, delavirdine, efavirenz ...*

Their side effects are less numerous but just as serious as those of the preceding category: hepatic and digestive dysfunctions, severe exanthems (skin rashes), and mainly central nervous system problems related to sleep, mood and behavior which can go as far as psychosis generating suicidal thoughts.

One of these molecules, nevirapine, has been frequently incriminated as being particularly dangerous for newborn or about-to-be-born infants. This product spreads through all the tissues and dangerously crosses the hemato-encephalic and the placental barriers protecting the fetus. It is also found in breast milk.

ANTIVIRAL MEDICATION IS BENEFICIAL

Nevertheless, nevirapine is the spearhead of the antiretroviral treatments administered in Africa to pregnant HIV-positive women and thus to their infants!

The third category is called "protease inhibitors", known under the generic names of *ritonavir, indinavir, saquinavir, nelfinavir, amprenavir* ...

They prevent the enzymes known as proteases from fulfilling their function of assembling the new viral proteins, which leads to the formation of incomplete, and thus non-viable viral particles.

When these medications were introduced into the treatment of AIDS, they were considered a great advance in AIDS therapy. In fact, they are also fearsome poisons for the body. Proteases are essential enzymes, particularly for intestinal functions. Their inhibition leads to serious digestive problems.

The side effects of this family of antiretrovirals are equally numerous and partly match those of the other categories of drugs. However, certain disorders are specific:

- Problems linked to intestinal dysfunction such as diarrhea, flatulence and lesions of the digestive tract;
- Lipodystrophy which causes on the one hand a loss of fats in the face, buttocks and limbs, and on the other hand abdominal obesity and building up of fatty lumps on the chest and neck (buffalo hump).

These effects are very disabling, not only at the physiological level, but also at the social level (patients feel deformed and isolate themselves).

Before the arrival of protease inhibitors in the treatment of AIDS, David Rasnick, (a biochemist expert on the subject) attended a conference during which a presentation made a particular impact on him, although it didn't have any direct relationship with AIDS. It concerned the results of experiments carried out on mice from which one gene had been removed. Either the mothers were barren, or the baby mice were born perfectly normal.

But around the 26th day, all the mice died, one after the other. Autopsies showed that they died of hunger. Their intestines were totally destroyed and their immune system had collapsed, the disappearance of T and B lymphocytes being due to a massive destruction of thymus and spleen.

In fact, the gene removed by the scientists controlled, amongst other things, the synthesis of a protease named "cathepsine D", which is also found in man and is absolutely essential for life.

When intestinal problems first appeared in patients treated with anti-proteases, David Rasnick realized that the catastrophic experience of the genetically modified mice was reproducing itself in human guinea pigs. Protease inhibitors paralyzed cathepsine D in particular, causing similar damage.

The 90s saw the arrival of poly-therapies with the prescription of two medications at first, then three or four, chosen from among the categories mentioned above. As the side effects added up, the results were often disastrous, deaths occurring from heart attacks, strokes, renal or liver failures, and other causes.

Nevertheless, this type of treatment appeared much less dangerous than the previous single molecule regimen, because much lower doses were administered, with periods of treatment interruptions which limited cumulative toxic effects. This probably explains why numerous patients treated with triple-therapies have shown fewer side effects.

Researchers, however, continuously work to develop new molecules. This offers far more profitable business returns than any attempt to identify the real causes of AIDS!

We must point out, however, that in certain patients affected by severe opportunistic infections, with major digestive difficulties or pneumonia, triple-therapy often improves the clinical state of the patients in a rapid and fairly spectacular fashion.

Such observations have often been interpreted as proof of the causal relationship between HIV and AIDS. This interpretation is erroneous, because it was subsequently shown that certain anti-proteases have a marked antibiotic effect against *candida albicans* and *pneumocystis carinii*, i.e. germs very frequently re-

ANTIVIRAL MEDICATION IS BENEFICIAL

sponsible for severe opportunistic infections.

EMERGENCY TREATMENT

Anti-virals were initially prescribed only to severely ill AIDS patients. Then they were given to clinically asymptomatic persons, but in whom the number of T4 lymphocytes was considered too low. Following this, individuals in good health and non-immunodeficient were put under treatment on the basis that they were found "HIV-positive" in serological tests (including infants).

The next stage was to prescribe anti-virals to HIV-negative persons suspected of having "put themselves at risk". A treatment (called mini-therapy) was prescribed since 2003 to anybody afraid of a possible risky behavior. This is an emergency treatment, which has to be taken in the hours following the "risky behavior", the principle being to kill the virus following its entry into the body, therefore not giving it time to get into the cells.

In such "emergencies", a triple-therapy is prescribed for forty-eight hours by the hospital emergency doctor. Afterwards, a consultant continues with antiviral treatments for six months.

In a 2004 French daily paper, a patient talked about the emergency treatment that he had received:

> *"It's very restricting, and puts you out of action! I had no strength left, and could hardly stand up. But I don't regret it at all. It has maybe saved my life."*

In the same article, a hospital doctor from Toulon said:

> *"We can't guarantee the success of this triple-therapy100%, but we've clearly seen a reduction of 80% in the risk of being infected."*

How can anyone claim such statistics? What scientific method could ever prove that a treatment has been effective on a person, when nobody knows whether this person is actually infected?

However, the answer is clear! Statistically, 20% of the people who received the emergency treatment were later tested HIV-positive.

TREATMENTS WORSE THAN THE ILLNESS

Apparently, the scientific establishment has no better way of treating immunodeficient patients other than with immunosuppressor molecules, thus aggravating their state of health instead of improving it.

Consequently, we can understand the high mortality observed since the introduction of the first high-dosage antivirals (1987–1990) in the treatment of AIDS.

But there is much worse!

That patients are being treated by such debatable methods is already sufficiently embarrassing. But where the boundaries of cynicism were overstepped was when these dangerous drugs began to be prescribed to persons in perfect health, under the pretext that an HIV-positive serological test had classified them under the category of victims of an alleged "HIV" infection.

However, we will see in a later chapter that these tests have no value in the diagnosis of an infection by the so-called "HIV".

OTHER MEDICATIONS

Like all active medications, antibiotics have side effects, as the manufactures themselves mention in their leaflets. It is for this reason that they must be used as directed, as any misuse can have damaging consequences to the body in general, and the immune system in particular.

In fact, as their name indicates, antibiotics destroy life, a positive action when it comes to eradicating pathogenic bacteria, but which also leads to the destruction of certain healthy cells if the amount or duration of treatment are excessive.

Corticosteroids are used extensively in the treatment of numerous inflammatory illnesses.

Hemophiliacs take many medications, as well as other immunosuppressor agents, in order to prevent the development of antibodies against the coagulation factors with which they are treated.

The same applies to persons who receive organ transplants or blood transfusions.

However, this class of medication causes an atrophy of the lymphatic ganglions and a reduction in the number of circulating white cells (T and B lymphocytes, and monocytes).

THE POLITICO-PHARMACEUTICAL SCHEMING

The pharmaceutical laboratories spend colossal sums to ensure the promotion of their products, and in particular the extremely expensive antivirals.

They are great purveyors of advertisements, as much in the media for the general public as in specialized publications, but this is far from being their only means of communication.

Doctors are particularly courted. Their ongoing education is continually influenced by the pharmaceutical companies.

Many doctors regularly earn a substantial income from taking part in inquiries about the long-term effects of medications, and they are periodically invited to congresses, conferences, symposia and other information programs in countries generally situated – in the Tropics!

It is very difficult for the professional publications to escape the insidious control of the pharmaceutical firms, because of their advertising, which is such a considerable source of profit. These pharmaceutical firms with their excessive and powerful public relations channels are the main source of information destined for journalists. It's easy to understand why all the newspaper articles go in the same orthodox direction.

In France, the commission charged with authorizing medications marketing (AMM), was until recently composed of a majority of members linked to pharmaceutical firms (from 65% to 80%).

The law of July 1, 1998, which replaced the *"Agence du médicament"* by the *Afssaps* fixed this situation by barring members of its commissions from being connected with private industry. Nevertheless, we could question the soundness of the decisions made by this organization, since most clinical trials carried out on these medications are under the control of the pharmaceutical firms, who generously finance the hospital services in which these trials are carried out (several thousand euros for each human "guinea pig"...).

Moreover, numerous associations and NGOs in the so-called "fight against AIDS" are almost invariably heavily subsidized by the same pharmaceutical corporations, explaining their obstinate militancy in favor of the scaling up of the provision of antiviral therapies.

In North America, the situation is even more serious than in Europe, pharmaceutical companies being among the principal financial backers of the main political parties.

For example, see **table 2** that shows the donations made by pharmaceutical companies during the election campaign (from 1997 to 1999) which resulted in the victory of George Bush in 2000. This table is an extract from a document presented by Dr Robert Herron (October 2001). It is noticeable that the Republican Party received four times more donations than the Democratic Party.

Pharmaceutical firms	Donations to the Democratic Party (in US dollars)	Donations to the Republican Party (in US dollars)
Abbott Laboratories	0	166,250
Aventis	156,785	395,945
Bristol-Myers Squib	253,300	686,418
Eli Lilly	181,500	375,644
Glaxo Wellcome	55,250	477,875
Hoffmann-La Roche	20,000	100,525
Merck	0	102,825
Pfizer	175,000	979,496
Pharmacia-Upjohn	60,000	135,000
Schering-Plough	166,000	513,500
Total	1,067,835	3,993,478

Table 2: Contributions from antiviral manufacturers to the campaign budgets of the two major parties in the USA between 1997 and 1999.

Consequently, it is easy to understand why political leaders jealously protect the interests of the pharmaceutical industry.

On 30th April 2000, following a report made by the CIA, Bill Clinton declared the AIDS epidemic as "a major threat to the security of the United States". That fell perfectly into the plans of the World Bank, whose president had announced several days previously that he would give considerable financial support to fight AIDS in poor countries.

As a result, billions of extra dollars fell into the hands of the pharmaceutical companies.

All of this is reminiscent of the "war against cancer" declared by Richard Nixon in 1972, an operation which did cost taxpayers outrageous sums ... without any result.

LIE #5
HIV-POSITIVITY IS A SIGN OF HIV INFECTION

This lie is certainly the most iniquitous of all those which are denounced in this book, because it has made millions of people believe that they were ill and contagious.

It brings to mind Jules Romains' Doctor Knock, who said:

"*Every healthy man ignores he is sick*" ....

("Tout homme bien portant est un malade qui s'ignore")

In all the history of medical virology, the isolation of a virus and the demonstration of its link to the causality of a specific pathology were most often the result of laboratory experiments on cell cultures. It was almost never from direct microbial isolation from patients, with direct proof of transmission of the illness.

We need to go back to the beginning of the history of virology to find examples of isolation and direct transmission, for example with smallpox.

There were, however, examples of transmission by a-cellular filtrates, thanks to the use of special filters which clearly disproved the hypothesis according to which the transmission of an illness was due to cells or bacteria, since living cells and bacteria are far too large to cross the filters.

These cases are, historically, at the origin of the first virological discoveries.

The filtration methods ("ultra-filtration" as it is often called) were sufficiently sophisticated to permit the approximation of the size of the "viral" particles, which were the infectious transmission agents, agents which were called "filtering principles" ("*principes filtrants*"), simply to underline the fact that these particles were small enough to pass through the filters used to isolate them in the laboratory.

This data on the approximate dimension of the viruses would suggest that numerous viruses probably measure from 0.1 to 0.2 micrometers in diameter, these viral particles being unquestionably too small to be visible with an optical microscope. It was, therefore, necessary to wait for the development of electron microscopy with its resolution power one hundred times greater, to be able to directly see viruses and take precise measurements of their diameters.

Nevertheless, historically, it is by the simple and direct techniques of ultra-filtration that Peyton Rous at the Rockefeller Institute in New York demonstrated in 1911 the transmission "by a-cellular ultra-filtrates" of a specific type of cancer in chickens, postulating, without ever having seen it but with excellent scientific reasons, the existence and the carcinogenic property of the virus which bears his name, the Rous sarcoma virus, or RSV.

Forty years later, Charlotte Friend working at the Sloan Kettering Institute in New York, used the same technology of ultra-filtration to demonstrate another virus that transmits a form of leukemia to certain mice. It was only in 1955, that advanced electron microscopy techniques allowed Étienne de Harven, co-author of this book, to demonstrate the "Friend virus" in leukemic mice.

This incursion into the history of virology is not out of place in this book on AIDS for a simple reason: the Rous and the Friend viruses are both what we call today retroviruses, like "HIV". So all the scientific background from these old studies

HIV-POSITIVITY IS A SIGN OF HIV INFECTION

applies very directly to the critical analysis of current research on the hypothetical "HIV".

In modern infectious virology, evidence of isolation and infectivity was most frequently based on cell culture techniques carried out in microbiology laboratories, with electron microscopy arriving later to allow:

1. Characterization of the structure and of the exact dimensions of the viruses, and
2. Their classification within the general framework of virology.

No surprise therefore, that, at the Pasteur Institute in 1983, the announcement of the alleged isolation of "HIV" depended essentially on an erudite combination of cell culture methods and electron microscopy.

It was, indeed, after studying very complex and hyper-stimulated cell cultures that the team from the Pasteur Institute was able to announce, in 1983, the discovery of a viral agent "which could be implicated in the cause of AIDS". And it was from these same cell cultures, which Luc Montagnier acknowledged to represent "retroviral soups", that they began to identify proteins that were attributed to this virus in a totally arbitrary manner.

In fact, since the supposed "HIV" had never been either isolated or purified (and has never been ever since), one could not reasonably attribute a viral origin to those proteins found in these cultures. These scientific considerations do not hold much weight against the fortune and celebrity which reward those who perfect the development of alleged serologic tests for HIV.

Historically, Robert Gallo, who registered a patent in the same evening of the historic press conference of April 1984 announcing the discovery of a virus which was "probably" responsible for AIDS, released a sample of his culture to the Abbott Laboratories for the development of the first screening tests for "HIV".

Thereafter, Gallo had to share this gold mine with Luc Montagnier who had given him the original culture.

VIRAL DETECTION TESTS

There are several types of tests for the diagnosis of viral infections:

- **Indirect tests,** which don't detect the virus itself, but the presence in the patient's body of specific antibodies manufactured by their immune system against the virus.

    These antibodies are detected by means of immuno-enzymatic techniques, such as those referred to as "HIV-positivity tests" for AIDS:

- **Direct tests,** which highlight the virus or its components (antigens, genome) within the body, viral particles being directly visualized by electron microscopy;

- **Tests based on the infection** of certain cell cultures (in the laboratory), or of susceptible laboratory animals.

ANTIGENS AND ANTIBODIES

Antigens constitute all the foreign substances that are liable to cause the production of antibodies.

This generic term combines elements variable in form, size, organic or chemical origin (bacteria, viruses, cells, pollen, various proteins...)

Manufactured by certain cells (type B lymphocytes), antibodies are proteins whose function is to recognize and attach themselves to antigens in order to mark them, so that cells of the immune system, specialized in the elimination of these antigens, can track and destroy them in macrophages.

It is something like the role played by foresters when they mark certain trees to indicate to the loggers which to cut down.

"For each antigen there is a specific antibody" used to be the rule until it was noticed that antibodies could sometimes confuse their target and mark other, unrelated antigens.

Thus, the same antibody can mark several types of antigens, and the same antigen can be marked by several varieties of antibodies.

HIV-POSITIVITY IS A SIGN OF HIV INFECTION

This is usually referred to as immunological "cross reactions". The entire science of immunology is in fact based, most exclusively, on these two concepts: antigens and antibodies. An intriguing problem is that these two words have reciprocal definitions: one can hardly define an antigen without talking about antibodies, and one cannot define an antibody without talking about antigens. To base the whole science of immunology on two concepts that define each other would probably make René Descartes turn in his grave!

VIRAL PROTEINS

Today, virologists use genetic engineering tools and molecular biology techniques, mostly "biochemical markers", to identify a virus. They increasingly neglect the essential and direct controls available with electron microscopy.

These "markers" permit, in principle, the molecular identification of the virus. In the same manner, deciphering its genome allows the drawing up of a genetic identity map (let us state once again that the genome of the alleged "HIV", after more than twenty years of efforts, has not yet been firmly established !).

With different research teams failing to find the same antigen proteins in their cultures, it took years before a consensus was reached (more or less) and a dozen proteins accepted as being "typical" of "HIV".

In fact, only their presence in complex cultures (and again, not in all of them!) determined this selection.

What about the specificity of these alleged viral proteins?

According to the available evidence, it is non-existent, since proof of their viral origin is missing, simply because "HIV" has never been purified. On the contrary, certain of these proteins correspond to elements that have nothing to do with viruses, being most likely of cellular origin.

For example, the protein called p24 corresponds to the molecular weight of myosin, and p41 to that of actin.

However, actin and myosin are essential proteins of muscle cells, and are therefore found abundantly in the body.

A study published in 1990 in *Cancer Research* showed that

half of 144 tested dogs presented antibodies against one or several of the antigen proteins attributed to "HIV". However, dogs never had either HIV or AIDS!

RELIABILITY OF THE SEROLOGICAL TESTS

Sero-diagnostic tests are intended to detect the presence of antibodies in biological liquids, generally blood serum.

The different techniques used all share the same principle: to detect a reaction between microbial antigens and the antibodies of the patient directed against these antigens.

People wanting to know their serological status initially undergo a test called "evaluation", the most current of which is the *Elisa* type. Simple and affordable, it is reputed to have a high *sensitivity*, i.e. is able to detect precisely the presence of antibodies in "infected" people.

If Elisa is positive, the test should, in most countries, be repeated for verification. If it proves again positive, a third test will be carried out which is called "confirmation", generally of the *Western Blot* type which is claimed to possess a strong *specificity*, i.e. it is capable of detecting precisely the absence of antibodies in "non-infected" people. (The Western blot test is not used in the UK, where it is regarded as unreliable).

Before they were put on the market, these tests were evaluated under rather strange conditions:

- As we have just seen, there is no proof that the selected antigens come from a retrovirus called HIV;
- Phenomena of cross reaction do not allow confirmation that the reacting antibodies are specific to the antigens present in the test;
- And finally, most studies carried out by the manufacturing firms to validate their tests are, scientifically, highly questionable.

Moreover, in order to conclusively demonstrate the sensitivity of an "HIV test", it must be evaluated on the largest possible

HIV-POSITIVITY IS A SIGN OF HIV INFECTION

population of individuals unquestionably known to be carriers of the virus. Unfortunately, "HIV" being directly undetectable, such proofs have never been presented.

On the other hand, specificity research should have been carried out on a strictly virus-free control population. For the same reason as previously indicated, such proof is still missing. Moreover, the first evaluations of specificity were carried out on samples taken from anonymous blood donors.

POSITIVE HERE; NEGATIVE THERE

The *Western Blot* type of test is used to confirm HIV-positivity detected by one or two tests of the *Elisa* type. Therefore it is though to be a most reliable test.

A *Western Blot* test comprises ten aligned bands corresponding to ten proteins that have been defined as typically and exclusively related to "HIV".

An international consensus on diagnostic procedures has never been satisfactorily reached. Consequently, a person can be declared HIV-positive in certain countries where only two bands are required, while that same person would be regarded as negative in other countries where the legislation requires three or four bands .

So, depending on the country where you live, your same serum, analyzed under identical conditions, can show HIV-positive or negative results.

But there is another, even more intriguing question. Since the ten proteins used in the tests are all declared as being typical of "HIV", one could ask the two simple clashing questions :

- Why are two to four bands necessary when only one should be sufficient to diagnose the presence of the virus?

- Why are only two to four bands necessary when the presence of the whole virus implies the presence of all the ten proteins that are attributed to it, and therefore the reaction of all the ten bands of the test?

TEN LIES ABOUT AIDS

FALSE POSITIVITY

Each of us possesses antibodies, the number and variety of which depend on aggression/infectious factors met during the course of our lives, our lifestyle, and even our race.

As David Rasnick, researcher specializing in protease inhibitors and active dissident against the official HIV thesis, rightly says:

> *"Different races have different ranges of naturally-occurring antibodies. That's why blacks have a nine times greater chance of testing positive than white Europeans, and a 33 times greater chance than Asians. It doesn't have anything to do with infection or health. In one study, a tribe of South American Indians was given Elisa tests. Thirteen percent of them tested HIV-positive, but nobody was sick. They just had antibodies that reacted with the test".*

As a matter of fact, these tests inspire so little confidence that in the United States the FDA (*Food and Drug Administration*) has not given its backing to any of them.

In addition, another mystery has not yet been elucidated: that of the dilution of the serum samples.

During the 90s, Dr Roberto Giraldo was working in a large university hospital laboratory in New York City. This gave him the opportunity to study the details of the serological tests routinely used for the diagnosis of AIDS.

The *Elisa* test particularly surprised him, because it was recommended by the manufacturers of the test to dilute the blood serum in the very high ratio of 1/400. This meant that it was necessary to take a small quantity of serum and dilute it 400 times with a thinner specially supplied by the manufacturer, a thinner which contained, amongst other things, bovine and calf serum as well as a lysate of human T lymphocytes!

Giraldo was surprised by this high initial dilution, since the majority of serological tests use almost pure serum. Certainly, in order to avoid certain risks of false positives, some tests require dilution, but the largest recommended until then (that relative to the detection of *cytomegalovirus*) was only 1/20.

HIV-POSITIVITY IS A SIGN OF HIV INFECTION

Incidentally, the other leading test, the *Western Blot*, also requires a strong dilution of 1/50.

Giraldo then asked himself in what way "HIV" was so different, from other microorganisms tested by comparable serological procedures, to necessitate such high dilution. He redid a group of tests that had proved negative, by using instead pure serums. They all tested "positive"! He obtained the same result on one hundred samples, even with his own blood serum.

Two explanations had to be considered: either the whole world possessed a more or less large titer of antibodies against "HIV", or the tests lacked specificity.

After having analyzed the problem from various angles, and having carried out other tests at intermediate dilutions, he logically concluded that most positive results were in fact false positives.

The *Elisa* is not the only problematic test. A study published in 1988 in the *Journal of American Medical Association* had already denounced the fact that the same blood sample sent to nineteen different laboratories for testing by means of the *Western Blot* had produced nineteen different results!

It is important to repeat that, because of the lack of an international standard, patients can be diagnosed HIV positive or negative according to which country they live in. Out of the ten test bands which *Western Blot* counts, two are sufficient in order to be judged "positive" and declared infected in Africa. In Great Britain it would need three, and four in Australia.

More embarrassingly, the tests have such a questionable specificity that the manufacturers themselves state that they cannot be used to confirm or disprove the presence of "HIV". They also state that there are a number of possible sources of false positives. Actually, back in 1996, sixty distinct medical conditions were documented as liable to confer "seropositivity". The list includes (See C. Johnston, under References):

- multiparity;
- hemophilia, blood transfusion;
- cancers;

- liver diseases (hepatitis, cirrhosis);
- tuberculosis;
- paludism (malaria);
- leprosy;
- recent vaccination (flu, hepatitis B, tetanus…);
- fever;
- auto-immune illnesses;
- hyperlipemia (presence of excessive lipids in the blood);
- treatment with gammaglobulins (preventative protection against infectious diseases;
- interferon treatments;
- renal failure (with or without hemodialysis);
- upper respiratory infections (cold, flu);
- herpes simplex I and II infections;
- organ transplant;
- rheumatoid polyarthritis;
- some auto-immune diseases;
- viral and mycobacterial infections;
- having already had false positives with other tests;
- etc...

THE VIRAL LOAD

The concept of "viral load" was introduced in the United States by Dr David Ho, also a promoter of multi-therapies, to explain the fact that nobody could find "HIV" directly in any patient. Dr Ho suggested that the virus knew how to make itself undetectable, but that it could be brought to light thanks to the PCR (*polymerase chain reaction*) technique, which is a process of amplification of DNA, that can allegedly measure what was de-

HIV-POSITIVITY IS A SIGN OF HIV INFECTION

scribed as the "viral load".

In 1997, David Ho and his colleagues treated a group of twenty patients with a bi-therapy combining AZT and protease inhibitor. When treatment began, the so-called "viral load" of these patients fell to an undetectable level and remained so. This result was claimed as evidence that the prescribed bi-therapy was effective, and Dr Ho quickly became a media personality (elected "Man of the Year 1996" by *Time Magazine*).

According to some orthodox scientists themselves, at least 99.8% of the retroviruses measured by the viral load test are not infectious!

Where do they come from? Are they incompletely formed particles? These dubious viruses, as well as those presented as virulent, have never been seen through an electron microscope. However, given the large quantity of particles claimed to be present in "high viral load" patients, nothing would have been easier.

During an historic international conference on AIDS, held in Pretoria in May 2000 at the invitation of the President of the Republic of South Africa, Mr. Thabo Mbeki, one of the authors of this book (ÉDH), clearly underlined the fact that, even using blood from patients labeled as having a high "viral load", nobody had ever managed to see through an electron microscope any retroviral particle in such samples. This assertion has never been contradicted.

Actually, if DNA molecules are detected in the viral load tests, they most likely originate from various cell debris present in the blood, and not from viral particles that nobody has ever seen.

It has been scientifically established that the human genome contains about 2% (or more) "sequences" of retroviral origin.

Therefore, the alleged "viral" load is easily explained by the presence of fragments of cell chromosomes, probably originating from disrupted leucocyte nuclei. It does not permit to demonstrate the hypothetical presence of particles of "HIV" in the blood.

Dr David Rasnick, previously mentioned, explains the mistake very well (extract from his interview with Celia Farber in *Gear* magazine):

> *"'Viral load' is the most powerful microscope ever developed,"* he says. *If the only way you can see something is by using the most powerful microscope, how clinically relevant can it be? If a person had real viremia you wouldn't need PCR to see it. Here you're talking about a level of about one virus particle in a drop of blood!*
>
> *Here's an example. When they look for HIV in breast milk, they do 45 cycles of PCR, which is a 35-trillion- fold amplification, in order to find enough genetic material. We are at the level of sensitivity of nuclear physics now with this PCR stuff. And David Ho talks about making HIV "undetectable"? It starts out undetectable. That's the whole point. HIV has always been more or less undetectable.*
>
> *So they've taken a number that is next to nothing, and mass multiplied it. But it's still next to nothing. Just a bunch of numbers that are used to scare people and make people go on these drugs.*
>
> *All this stuff about wanting to get to zero, or to undetectable, is absurd because it implies that a single particle of HIV is lethal, but it's not.*
>
> *This is the biological equivalent of counting bumpers in a junk-yard and saying they represent functional cars."*

Moreover, the inventor of the PCR technique, Dr Kary Mullis (who won the Nobel Prize for Chemistry in 1993 for this invention), regards the use of PCR for an alleged measurement of a hypothetical "viral load" as fraudulent. This brilliant scientist is, however, banging his head against a brick wall. His protests about the abuse of his invention are ignored.

AFRICA: A SPECIAL CASE

Numerous infections, and particularly those which are endemic in Africa, are the source of numerous false positive HIV tests.

For example, a study carried out in central Africa showed that tuberculosis and leprosy probably account for 70% of the false positives observed in these areas.

HIV-POSITIVITY IS A SIGN OF HIV INFECTION

Moreover, problems of insufficient infrastructure and limited budget have made the use of *Elisa* testing in Africa very difficult. Consequently, in 1985, the WHO recommended a set of clinical criteria that may support the diagnosis of AIDS in the absence of serological evidence. This recommendation was made at a conference held in Bangui and is therefore referred to as the "Bangui definition" for the diagnosis of AIDS in African patients.

This definition takes into account two types of symptoms classified according to their importance:

The major signs:

- weight loss greater than 10%
- chronic diarrhea lasting at least one month
- persistent or intermittent fever lasting at least one month

The minor signs:

- persistent cough for at least one month
- generalized itching
- cutaneous herpes
- other chronic and scattered *herpes simplex* infections
- oro-pharyngeal candida
- lymphadenopathy (swelling of the lymphatic ganglions)

However, the clinical symptoms listed in the "Bangui definition" are so common in tropical medicine as to make the resulting epidemiological data devoid of any real significance.

The other method used for statistical studies within the African population is no more scientifically convincing.

Estimates made by ONUSIDA and WHO are done by the *"Sentinelle"* method, which consists of counting the number of pregnant HIV-positive women frequenting health clinics, and in acrobatically extrapolating these numbers to estimate the prevalence of "HIV" in entire populations!

These statistical methods have been severely criticized (See James Chin's 2007 book, under References), primarily because multiparity is a known cause of false positive HIV tests. Unfortunately, the critics have not managed to shake the confidence expressed by the WHO authorities in their methods.

In addition, if the tests carried out are of the *Western Blot* type, two bands are sufficient to establish HIV-positivity in Africa, against three or four bands in Western countries. This obviously makes any epidemiological comparison extremely uncertain.

As the statistical studies are only related to pregnant women, how is it possible to know the rate of HIV-positivity in the other women, in children, and in men?

Here again, the figures obtained are extrapolated in a dangerously arbitrary way, statistical evaluations being based on models that were frequently changed (See Rian Malan, under References). Decidedly, one may wonder whether statistics can sometimes represent the worst form of lie!

The data summarized in this chapter shows that the so-called HIV-positive tests fail to provide any scientifically acceptable evidence proving alleged HIV infections.

For twenty years, that lie has had tragic consequences. Millions of individuals were led to believe that a positive test meant the diagnosis of an illness, when it simply indicates a high antibody titer. They were equally led to believe that they were contagious when they didn't carry any recognizable virus. Finally, they were also led to believe that they were destined for an early death. All of that has resulted in a dramatic increase in the numbers of exclusions, depressions, societal havocs, suicides, and very frequently serious medicinal poisoning (AZT), often lethal with the doses used at the start of the so-called epidemic!

LIE #6
AIDS IS CONTAGIOUS

Symptoms of all sexually transmitted diseases (syphilis, gonorrhea, genital or anal herpes), are evident several days after transmission, in all patients and without any distinction between individuals.

But in the case of HIV, it will take months or years before the alleged AIDS virus will express its hypothetical pathogenicity. Moreover, this virus seems to infect only a very restricted category of individuals.

In addition, in classic infections specific microorganisms can usually be isolated or cultured directly from the patients, while the AIDS virus is only detectable on the basis of alleged molecular "markers", which are non-specific.

HOMOSEXUALS AND AIDS

The first five cases of AIDS were observed and described in Los Angeles in 1981. The author of this initial report, Michael Gottlieb, had clearly indicated that the five patients were homosexuals, and were all using amyl nitrite (poppers). Also, he stressed the fact that the five patients had never met and could not therefore have contaminated each other.

TEN LIES ABOUT AIDS

What made Michael Gottlieb think that he had just discovered a new infectious illness? There is no answer to this question, and the mystery remains complete.

A parable may help understanding better the importance of the question: let us imagine that a doctor looks after the health of a hundred workers who are all working in an old dye factory, badly ventilated, and where air pollution with plenty of lead salts is obvious. After a few years, the doctor identifies a dozen cases of lead poisoning among these workers. Will that doctor conclude that lead poisoning is a contagious disease simply because these workers all worked in the same factory? Or will he rather conclude that his patients have all been inhaling the same toxic lead salt, and as a result have all developed the same pathology?

The answer is obvious ...

How can we explain that Gottlieb did not reason in the same fashion, and did not immediately understand that his five patients had all been exposed to the same toxic drugs (mostly amyl nitrite), and as a result had all developed the same pathology?

Another observation, equally important, should have cast serious doubt upon the infectious hypothesis from the start: almost all the patients were men, and the disease was initially referred to as "GRID", standing for Gay Related Immune Deficiency. In fact, all the reports relating to what was rapidly called an epidemic showed that 90% to 95% of the patients were male.

Here again, no surprise! No question asked about this most unusual epidemiological phenomenon!

But never mind, the hypothesis of the contagiousness of AIDS was well on its way, and it was necessary to keep it going at all costs, even if it was necessary to believe that "HIV" only attacked men!

Because "HIV" research was becoming big business in the United States, demands for an enormous government research budget was made.

However, when patients were exclusively homosexual and/or IV drug users, their number wasn't high enough to justify astronomical research grants.

As New York journalist Celia Farber rightly remarked in an

article that appeared as early as 1992, that, for the establishment, it was urgent to create panic amongst as great a number of people as possible, preferably the entire population. From this devilish strategy originated the "invention" of heterosexual AIDS!

And when members of Congress of the United States started to worry ("Look out man: this terrible illness could get you too!"), then voting huge budgets became easy, and dollars began raining down... And are still raining down today...

HETEROSEXUAL AIDS

In the summer of 1987, a colossal media campaign of highly biased information commenced with the aim of plunging the heterosexual community into panic.

"Everybody can catch AIDS!" That was the essence of the message sent by the health authorities in the USA, a message relayed with complete servility by the media, worldwide.

There was a sudden rush to the screening centers...

Positive tests, as one would expect, amounted to thousands among people leading a conventional lifestyle.

The name "GRID" was promptly forgotten, as unacceptably discriminative. It was substituted with the name "AIDS" that was more fitting to plunge the entire population into panic.

"We told you so!" trumpeted public health officials, who arrogantly announced that the new plague would create catastrophic ravages throughout the entire world population.

How had the virus jumped from the at-risk groups to spread into the general population? Perhaps via bi-sexual men?

The only recommended way to escape from contamination was sexual abstinence or possibly the use of a condom.

"HIV" was initially believed to be transmitted through blood. Now it was necessary to beware of other carriers like sperm, saliva, vaginal secretions and even sweat.

The phobia about infection was such that everybody began to mistrust everybody else. Everybody who had tested HIV-positive became untouchable, ostracized from social life, rejected everywhere, often by their own family. Some children were expelled from schools.

TEN LIES ABOUT AIDS

On their side, the prophets of doom, preachers in innumerable churches and sects prevailing in the USA, did not hold back from announcing that AIDS was God's punishment for humans living uninhibited sex lives.

"Is your baby HIV-positive? Shame on you, unworthy parents." That was the kind of sermon occasionally heard at the time.

This wind of panic was also blowing in Europe, and then throughout the whole world. Those who were around at that time recall: the work colleagues who fled the plague victim; the companies that sacked the immoral; the friends who didn't call any more; the finger pointed at parents for having created a monster; spouses who were divorced; and the breach of contract by the employers of he or she who had deliberately caught the virus during extra-marital sexual relations...

From that moment, enormous sums were devoted to informing the public about risky behavior, publicizing the need to use condoms, and setting up exchange programs for sterile syringes.

Very recently (2007) however, Dr. James Chin, formerly Chief of the Surveillance Unit of the Global Program on AIDS (GPA) of WHO, Geneva, Switzerland, published a book entitled "The Aids Pandemic – The collision of epidemiology with political correctness". Chin has considerable authority on matters of AIDS epidemiology, and definitely belongs to the mainstream (i.e. non-dissident!) group of AIDS researchers. Still, in the introduction of his book, he states:

> *"My HIV/AIDS paradigm is that epidemic HIV transmission requires human behaviors that involve having unprotected sex with multiple and concurrent sex partners and/or routinely sharing needles and syringes with other injecting drug users (IDU). According to my understanding of HIV transmission dynamics, HIV epidemics cannot occur in populations where high risk patterns and the highest prevalence of such risk behaviors are not present. Exaggeration of the potential for HIV to spread into the "general" population is a "glorious" myth perpetuated by UNAIDS, AIDS program advocates, and activists, partly to avoid further stigmatization of persons with the highest levels of HIV risk behaviors. UNAIDS also wants the public and policy*

AIDS IS CONTAGIOUS

makers to be fearful about HIV infections "jumping out" from these foci of infection to spread into the "general population". Yet no such spread into the general population has occurred!" And somewhat later: "This myth of a high potential for "generalized" HIV epidemics has resulted in a large and unnecessary amount of effort and funds being used for programs directed to the general population and specially youths. Yet these groups, outside sub-Saharan Africa, are at minimal to NO RISK of acquiring HIV from risky sexual behaviors".

Chin's statements are in total conflict with the current dogma obviously inspiring UNAIDS policies. It is practically minimizing down to zero the risk of HIV heterosexual transmission in the general population.

However, to better demonstrate that AIDS is actually not an infectious disease (and is therefore not transmissible), the different carriers alleged to be HIV transmitters must be analyzed.

TRANSMISSION BY SPERM

According to official studies, the demonstration of transmission of AIDS by sperm is not conclusive at all.

In 1991, a study published in the medical journal *Fertility and Sterility* showed that out of twenty-eight male HIV-positive subjects, only four had traces of "HIV" (in fact, traces of enzymatic activity erroneously attributed to a retrovirus) in their sperm. In a previous study, the proportion was one in twelve.

All the studies carried out never showed more than 28% to 30% of so-called "contaminated" sperm samples, and the authors are only talking of one to ten copies per ejaculation, which is one virus per million of spermatozoa.

AIDS experts themselves agree that such a quantity is insufficient to transmit infection. Despite that, they continue to claim that sperm is a contaminating carrier.

AIDS IN PRISON

It is often claimed that AIDS is particularly widespread in prisons, given the promiscuity and the need to assuage sexual desire in the absence of female company.

The rate of HIV-positivity is detected by means of serological tests. In fact, the majority of HIV-positives were found among the drug-addicted prisoners. Sexual promiscuity has nothing to do with alleged secondary infections among prisoners. This is borne out in a letter published in the *British Medical Journal* of 26th January 2002, by Dr Stuart W Dwyer, a doctor in a South African prison, a country where prisons are over-populated (often up to thirty prisoners in a cell), where homosexuality is widespread, and where the use of condoms is practically non-existent.

According to the viral hypothesis, prisons should be favorable to the spread of AIDS, since real sexually transmitted diseases (STDs) are frequently observed there.

In the prison where Dr Dwyer works, all prisoners with an STD are tested for "HIV", as are also those with any other illness not cured after two weeks. However, it has been found that the rate of HIV-positivity among prisoners has varied between 2% and 4% over seven years of testing, and that over the same period only two deaths could be attributed to AIDS, out of a population of 550 prisoners.

It is acknowledged that the average rate of HIV-positivity throughout all South African prisons is 2.3%. One could therefore expect that the prevalence should be far lower in the general population than in prisons where all the conditions are met for the propagation of contagious illnesses.

Very surprisingly, however, all official estimates supplied by the World Health Organization (WHO) give a rate of HIV-positivity in the neighborhood of 20% for the whole South African population. Later, we will see how WHO comes up with their most alarming estimates.

AIDS AND PROSTITUTION

Being obviously the group most exposed to sexually transmitted diseases, prostitutes pose a serious problem to the health authorities because AIDS is not spreading within this community. More precisely, it only affects those prostitutes who are intravenous drug addicts, sparing almost all the others.

AIDS IS CONTAGIOUS

Moreover, AIDS does not resemble any of the sexually transmitted diseases that all occur rapidly (in a few days), without distinction between race and sex, with the responsible microbe being readily detectable.

Supporters of the viral hypothesis never paid much attention to these inconsistencies, and they continue to propagate the idea that AIDS is transmitted by a heterosexual route, above all when sexual encounters have taken place with prostitutes.

However, studies carried for many years give a completely different perspective. For example, in New Jersey (a State where drug abuse is particularly rampant) a study carried out on a group of 62 prostitutes diagnosed as HIV-positive showed that 47 of them (76%) were intravenous drug abusers. Out of the remaining 15, the investigators suspected that many of them had lied and were also using drugs, while others had recently been affected by infectious illnesses (likely representing sources of false positives).

Another study carried out in Nevada on 535 prostitutes did not find a single case of HIV-positivity. On the other hand, at the same time, they found 6% positive tests among prostitutes incarcerated in Nevada prisons, all of whom were drug addicts.

Other studies were carried out in Europe:

- Paris: no HIV-positivity among the 56 prostitutes tested;
- London: again, not a single one among 50 prostitutes tested in a specialized STD clinic;
- Nuremberg: no HIV-positivity among 339 listed prostitutes;
- in Italy, only the drug-addicted prostitutes were shown to be HIV-positive.

A shocking example of biased and obstinate interpretation of clinical data appears in a study published in *The Lancet* of 16th November 1996. A group made up of Kenyan and Canadian researchers had followed over a dozen years (from 1985 to 1994) a group of 424 prostitutes working in Nairobi, Kenya.

TEN LIES ABOUT AIDS

Despite numerous sexual relations (without condoms), 43 of these prostitutes remained HIV-negative in tests, viral load included. Rather than casting doubt on the sexually transmissible nature of AIDS, and rather than implicating drug addiction and malnutrition (both very widespread) in those who became HIV-positive during the study, researchers concluded that a certain proportion of individuals "highly exposed to the virus" must have developed some natural protection making them resistant to HIV infection!

MOTHER TO CHILD TRANSMISSION

The birth of a child is a miracle of nature, a symbol of the triumph of life.

Health authorities directed the anathema towards mothers who dared bring babies into the world when they were HIV-positive.

How could these mothers possibly "infect" their offspring?

Theoretically, in three ways: during the fetal life, during birth, and by breast-feeding.

Neither of these alleged modes of "Mother to child" (MTC) transmission has received the slightest level of scientific support. More specifically, to incriminate breast-feeding, one would expect evidence for the presence of retroviral particles in breast milk from seropositive mothers. Such evidence is totally missing. It has never been possible to convincingly demonstrate retroviral particles by electron microscopy directly in breast milk.

A report published in 1985 (See L. Thiry, under reference), however, states the contrary. This report was based on the identification of surrogate molecular markers in complex cell culture systems; it should be criticized exactly on the same grounds as the pretended "isolation" of HIV, at the Pasteur Institute in 1983, which was reviewed in Chapter 2. One can no more detect the virus in the newborn than in the mother. The only "evidence" to the contrary is exclusively based on surrogate, highly questionable laboratory testing.

We know that antibodies circulating in the body of a very young child are those of his/her mother. The child starts to produce its own antibodies, progressively replacing maternal antibodies over a period of a few months.

It is no surprise, therefore, that the antibody tests which have given a positive reaction for the mother will produce identical results in the newborn. With no treatment, these children become naturally HIV-negative in the majority of cases.

In spite of all these facts, health authorities continue, nevertheless, to advise and forcefully insist on giving antivirals to such infants, likely exposing them to considerable toxic damage (See Liam Scheff, under References).

A French team published a study that is exemplary of the state of mind of some researchers who are fully determined to prove, against all logical analysis, that the AIDS virus exists.

This study was published in the *New England Journal of Medicine* of 22nd June 1999 (Volume 320 – No. 25) and is signed by a group of researchers from the Necker Hospital in Paris.

Here is a summary of the résumé, published as a leading article:

> *"Assessment of the risks of transmission of infection with human immunodeficiency virus type 1 (HIV-1) from mother to newborn is difficult, partly because of the persistence for up to a year of maternal antibodies transmitted passively to the infant. To determine the frequency of prenatal transmission of HIV infection, we studied from birth 308 infants born to seropositive women, 62 percent of whom were intravenous drug abusers. Of 117 infants evaluated 18 months after birth, 32 (27 percent) were seropositive for HIV or had died of the acquired immunodeficiency syndrome (AIDS) (n = 6); of the 32, only 2 remained asymptomatic. Another 76 infants (65 percent) were seronegative and free of symptoms, whereas 9 (8 percent) were seronegative but had symptoms suggestive of HIV-1 infection. The infants infected with HIV-1 did not differ from the others at birth with respect to weight, height, head circumference, or rate of malformations, but as compared with newborns who were seronegative at 18 months, their serum IgM levels were higher (78 +/- 81 mg per deciliter vs. 38 +/- 39 mg per deciliter; P less than 0.03) and their CD4 lymphocyte counts were lower (2054 +/- 1221 per cubic millimeter vs. 2901 +/- 1195 per cu-*

bic millimeter; P less than 0.006). Neither maternal risk factors nor the route of delivery was a predictor of seropositivity at 18 months; however, 5 of the 6 infants who were breast-fed became seropositive, as compared with 25 of 99 who were not (P less than 0.01). We conclude that approximately one third of the infants born to seropositive mothers will have evidence of HIV-1 infection or of AIDS by the age of 18 months, and that about one fifth of this group will have died."

Surprisingly, in a cohort of 308 children followed since their birth, only 117 are left 18 months later. The statistical disappearance of the 191 others is not explained!

Moreover, 62% of the mothers were intravenous drug addicts. It would have been interesting to know what was the behavior of the remaining 38% with regard to other drugs, to malnutrition, to alcoholism, to medication abuse, etc.

Then, almost as an anecdote, we are told that nine HIV-negative children nevertheless had AIDS symptoms, but this doesn't seem to have posed any problem to the authors of the study.

Moreover, the rate of IgM (M-type immunoglobulins, antibodies) was higher in HIV-positive individuals. This was to be expected since HIV-positivity simply signals that the tested individual is a carrier of numerous antibodies of diverse origin, without any need for those raised against an elusive retrovirus.

The number of CD4 (T4) in HIV-positives was found less than that in HIV-negatives. The tables indicate the average CD4 numbers, followed by the observed margins. Consequently, numerous HIV-negative children had CD4 counts inferior to those of HIV-positives. Average counts are informative but individual cases cannot be ignored.

Finally, the last-but-one paragraph suggests that breastfed children had a three times greater risk of being HIV-positive than those fed with "formula", evidently encouraging the sale of industrial products.

In fact, it is natural that a breastfed child receives the antibodies of its mother at the same time as nutritive substances, making mother's milk irreplaceable. Far from being dangerous to the child, those antibodies participate in building up its im-

AIDS IS CONTAGIOUS

mune defenses.

This study is also deficient on essential case histories of the patients. It does not mention any possible immunosuppressor factors (for example, serious malnutrition or antiviral treatments) that could account for AIDS (and sometimes death) of certain HIV-positive children.

The dogmatic tune is heard throughout this paper: "*HIV-positives can only die of 'HIV' infections*".

The conclusion of this chapter on lie number 6 is that, reviewing critically all the scientifically available evidence, AIDS is quite clearly not a contagious disease. The clinical reality of AIDS is totally indisputable, and the syndrome has opened a most dramatic page in the history of contemporary medicine. However, there is simply no way the syndrome can be scientifically classified as a sexually transmissible disease.

That being said, it remains obvious that real and well-known sexually transmissible diseases like syphilis, gonorrhea, or herpes are very serious public health concerns which call for widespread and continuing public education efforts, aiming at all possible modes of prevention including the use of condoms.

LIE #7
HIV CAUSES NUMEROUS ILLNESSES

The measles virus is only found in people with measles, the flu virus only in people suffering from flu, etc.

With "HIV", a new era began: that of multi-potent viruses, capable of causing a wide variety of infectious diseases (due to immunodeficiency), and also pathologies ("AIDS indicator diseases") having nothing to do with the immune system.

In all, there are thirty illnesses said to be caused by this multi-directional killer. Surprisingly, however, biologists and health professionals readily accepted such multiple pathogenicity, in spite of the fact that it brought into question all that they had previously learned!

Their ability to critically evaluate the data was probably impaired by eloquent and politically correct presentations made by a few prominent laboratory heads and/or by leaders of pharmaceutical companies. Obviously, once you become part of some new scientific elite, you can present the craziest hypothesis and be certain to receive a large public audience, thanks to the media's constant search for fear- generating sensationalism. Scientific demonstrations are somehow not necessary; being famous is enough.

Every age has the gods it deserves.

Three main types of illnesses are thought to indicate HIV in-

fection :
- the viral, bacterial or fungal infections called "opportunists". These are the most common;
- some cancers, lymphomas and Kaposi's sarcomas;
- certain diseases called "linked to HIV".

Contrary to popular belief, nearly two-thirds of the people counted as being infected with HIV in the developed countries are not ill. It is sufficient to be tested as HIV-positive, and to have less than 200 CD4 T-lymphocytes per mm^3 of blood to enter, quite automatically, in the world's AIDS statistics.

As an example, **table 3** gives an idea of the frequency of the most current illnesses associated with AIDS. It relates to cases appearing in the United States in 1997, the last year for which the CDC published this type of statistic. Registered cases of AIDS totaled 60,161. This table is adapted from that published by Duesberg, Koehnlein and Rasnick in the *Journal of Biosciences* of June 2003, already mentioned.

INFECTIOUS DISEASES

In cases of immune deficiency, the body can no longer effectively control some microorganisms which, therefore, attack defenseless individuals in an "opportunistic" manner.

Susceptibility to infectious diseases results from immuno-deficiency no matter what the origin of the deficiency is. In cases of AIDS, the majority of the opportunistic infections involve fungi, yeasts or mycobacteria. However, in nature, these organisms may function in the recycling of biological material acting primarily on dead tissues.

Specific remarks on AIDS associated infectious diseases are as follows.

HIV CAUSES NUMEROUS ILLNESSES

Illnesses	Method of diagnosis	Number of cases	Percentage of total
No illness	Number of T4 less than 200 per mm3 + HIV-positivity	36,634	60.9%
Microbial illnesses	Pneumocystosis	9,145	15.2%
	Candidiasis	3,846	6.4%
	Tuberculosis and mycobacterial infections	3,537	5.9%
	Cytomegalovirus infections	1,138	2.7%
	Pneumonia	1,347	2.2%
	Herpes virus infections	1,250	2.1%
	Cryptococcal infections	1,168	1.9%
	Toxoplasmosis	1,073	1.8%
Non-microbial illnesses	Weight loss	4,212	7%
	Kaposi's sarcoma	1,500	2.5%
	Dementia	1,409	2.3%
	Lymphomas - Leukemias	850	1.4%
	Cancer of the uterus and cervix	144	0.2%

Table 3: *Frequency of appearance of AIDS illnesses in the United States for the year 1997. Total number of cases: 60,161.*

- **PNEUMOCYSTOSIS**

Pneumocytis carinii pneumonia, or PCP, is so typical of AIDS that it was almost synonymous with it at the beginning of the 80s, being by far the most frequent serious infection found among homosexual and drug-addicted patients (two-thirds of the cases in the USA).

The responsible microorganism, *pneumocyctis carinii*, had

been considered for a long time as a protozoa, but is now included among a group of fungal agents. It is very widespread throughout the world, and harmless under normal circumstances.

In western countries, 90% of the population are carriers of anti-bodies against *pneumocyctis carinii*, which indicates that they have been in contact with the germ without developing pneumonia.

Pneumocystosis is therefore the opportunistic illness *par excellence*, because it only develops in individuals with a weakened immune system.

"HIV" has been blamed for causing this immunodeficiency. However, it has been known since the 30s that it is rampant in certain premature newborns, in people suffering from malnutrition, in the cases where corticosteroids are administered (experiments dating from the 50s), or following anti-cancer chemotherapy.

- **TUBERCULOSIS**

Together with malaria, this is the most widespread infectious disease in Africa, and generally very common in under-developed countries. However, it only became one of the "AIDS" indicator diseases in 1993. Its inclusion in the list caused an explosion in the "infection" statistics, above all in Africa.

The responsible microorganism is a mycobacteria, *mycobacterium tuberculosis*, discovered by the German microbiologist Robert Koch, in 1882.

Although a small rise has been noted in the last few years, tuberculosis has almost disappeared from developed countries, since its prevalence in the western population is less than 0.5 per 1,000 (0.2 per 1,000 in France). It is still observed among drug-addicts, chronic alcoholics and people living in impoverished circumstances.

Tuberculosis, however, remains endemic in developing countries, where 95% of the cases are found. It is the most deadly infectious disease in the world (about 2 million deaths each year).

HIV CAUSES NUMEROUS ILLNESSES

The ten countries most affected are: India, China, Indonesia, Bangladesh, Pakistan, Nigeria, Philippines, Republic of South Africa, Ethiopia and Vietnam.

Most surprisingly, however, in 1991 the international health authorities attributed a large majority of cases of tuberculosis to HIV, which automatically, and considerably increased the already alarming numbers of deaths "due to HIV".

Since the beginning of medical history, tuberculosis has been rampant among populations suffering from malnutrition and living in deplorable sanitary conditions.

The upsurge in cases of tuberculosis in poor countries is not the result of the harmful effect of any virus. It results from progressive and continual deterioration in socio-economic conditions, incessant wars, as well as the incredible incompetence of the international organizations that are meant to help underprivileged populations.

Instead, these organizations prefer to flood these territories with vaccines and antiviral medicines, rather than giving these destitute people drinking water and elementary sanitary equipment.

In developing countries, HIV-positive tuberculosis patients are reported as AIDS cases. On the other hand, HIV-negative tuberculosis patients are simply reported as TB patients, or not reported at all.

Why the difference? The reason is simply because reporting AIDS cases brings in millions of dollars from major international agencies, while reporting TB cases brings in close to nothing.

- **OTHER PULMONARY INFECTIONS**

Recurring pneumonia (from *mycobacterium*, pneumococcal or *hemophilus*) and interstitial pneumonia (from *cytomegalovirus*) have also been reported.

- **CANDIDIASIS**

There are several types of candidiasis. The most common is oro-pharyngeal disease (thrush), but esophageal, pulmonary and genital forms have also been reported. These infections are characterized by the presence of a yeast, *candida albicans*. Affected areas become very painful, and the patient finds it difficult to swallow.

Candidiasis appears at least once in all AIDS patients.

This is not surprising because it is frequently observed in immunodeficient subjects, for example after antibiotic or corticosteroid treatment, in women taking contraceptive pills or hormone replacement therapy, in drug-addicts, in cases of stress, and following chemical poisoning ...

- **CEREBRAL TOXOPLASMOSIS**

This type of encephalitis is characterized by the presence of intra-cerebral abscess caused by a protozoan (small unicellular micro-organisms), *toxoplasma gondii*. This parasite is widespread throughout the world. For example, 70% of the French population possesses antibodies directed against it.

Under normal circumstances, toxoplasmosis is harmless (except in pregnant women when there is a possible contamination of the fetus). On the other hand, it is dangerous in immunodeficient subjects.

In France, about a quarter of AIDS patients develop this disease (5% in the USA), with a mortality rate in the neighborhood of 25%.

The infection primarily affects the central nervous system (brain) but can equally affect heart, lungs, liver or eyes.

Principal symptoms are feverish headaches, somnolence, loss of orientation, epileptic seizures and paralysis.

Although classified as one of the neurological signs of AIDS, toxoplasmosis is, obviously, an opportunistic infection.

- **CRYPTOCOCCOSIS**

This meningitis is caused by a microscopic yeast, *cryptococcus neoformans*. It is characterized by a meningeal syndrome (intense headache amplified by noise and light) plus a certain mental confusion (loss of spatio-temporal awareness), behavioral troubles (agitation, aggressiveness) and extreme drowsiness.

If spreading occurs, the yeast can also affect the skin (producing a type of ulcerated lesion resembling acne).

If cerebral abscesses develop, symptoms become identical to those of toxoplasmosis. As with this latter, cryptococcosis is an opportunist infection.

- **INFECTIONS OF THE DIGESTIVE TRACT**

Numerous infections of the digestive tract can be either of bacterial (*salmonella, shigella, campylobacter…*), fungal (*mycobacterium, candida*), viral (*cytomegalovirus, herpes…*) or parasitic origin (*cryptosporidium, giardia, ameba, strongyloides…*).

Again, numbers of these microorganisms are present in many individuals without causing any problem. They can, however, cause diarrhea, anemia, fever and weight-loss in cases of immune deficiency.

- **SKIN COMPLAINTS**

These are equally numerous and varied. The most common is candidiasis, which has already been mentioned.

The fact that they are more frequent in AIDS cases than in the general population does not indicate any direct causal relationship with HIV. On the contrary, there is some reason to think that they are either the result of psychosomatic problems related to stress, or, more often, side effects of toxic treatments.

Here is a non-exhaustive list of observed skin disorders:

- Recurrent Herpes (cold sores, genital or anal herpes)
- Herpes Zoster (shingles)
- Hairy Leukoplakia of the tongue (whitish deposits on the edges of the tongue)
- Psoriasis (red lesions covered with whitish scales)
- Seborrheic Dermatitis (red scaly patches on the face and scalp
- Folliculitis (inflammation of the hair roots)

- Prurigo (localized spots on the skin causing intense itching)
- Impetigo
- Classic warts
- *Molluscum contagiosum* (small sub-cutaneous warts white or pink on face, neck, trunk, buttocks or genital organs)
- Ano-genital warts
- Xeroderma
- Eczema

- **CMV RETINITIS**

This is the origin of most common ophthalmic complaint in AIDS patients. It appears only in advanced stages of the illness and is caused by the presence of *cytomegalovirus,* CMV, a typically opportunistic herpes-like virus.

In the absence of appropriate treatment, the virus may destroy the entire retina, causing blindness.

- **PROGRESSIVE MULTI-FOCAL LEUCOENCEPHALITIS**

This disorder, occurring in about 4% of AIDS patients, and which is thought to be caused by reactivation of a human *papovavirus* (the JC virus) causes demyelination (destruction of the external coating of the nerve fibers) of the white matter of the brain.

It leads progressively to blindness, loss of speech and lack of coordination of movements, without any fever.

- **COCCIDIOIDOMYCOSIS**

Also known as "San Joaquin fever" this illness is endemic in South America, Central America and in the south-western part of the United States. It is caused by the inhalation of spores of a fungus called *Coccidioides immitis.*

In low risk patients the infection is benign and does not require treatment, but in immunodeficient subjects it causes acute

HIV CAUSES NUMEROUS ILLNESSES

respiratory distress which can be followed by osteo-articulatory and cerebro-meningeal disorders, the prognosis being very severe in AIDS patients, mortality exceeding 70%.

NEOPLASIAS

- **KAPOSI'S SARCOMA**

It was described for the first time in 1872 by Moritz Kaposi, in Austria. Rare cases had been observed in central Europe and in the Mediterranean area, in men aged from fifty to seventy. Since 1960, it has been suspected to be endemic in central Africa.

This disorder can hardly be classified as a typical cancer, because it is often reversible. In fact, its exact nature is not yet well understood.

It is characterized by an anarchic proliferation of cells covering the internal walls of blood vessels, and manifests itself by the appearance of purplish/brown red patches on the skin.

Lesions can spread in the digestive tract, as well as in the liver, lymphatic ganglions, lungs, and spleen.

Fifty percent of the patients die within a year.

In the 1970s, numerous cases of Kaposi's sarcoma (KS) were documented in patients suffering from iatrogenic immunodeficiency (i.e. caused by medication).

Before the advent of AIDS, cases were reported, in the USA, almost exclusively among homosexuals. It is often one of the first AIDS disorders to appear in homosexuals in large cities in the west, while their number of CD4 T-lymphocytes is still within norms. Furthermore, Kaposi's sarcoma equally affects serologically tested HIV-positives and HIV-negatives, which raises serious doubts about its retroviral infection origin.

In its classic form, Kaposi's sarcoma is primarily localized on the legs. But in AIDS affected individuals the lesions are mostly facial, involving in particular nose, mouth and palate. All practitioners know these localizations very well. And yet, they don't recognize (or don't want to recognize...) that these parts of the body are in direct contact with inhaled nitrites by users of "poppers".

That KS results from chemical cell poisoning of the blood vessels seems very likely, although herpesvirus type 8 has been suspected to be etiologically related. Other cases of Kaposi's sarcoma, outside of AIDS, are recorded in patients undergoing general corticoid or immuno-suppressor treatment following organ transplant.

Cancers of the lungs, uterus, testes and others have also been described as AIDS related, for no scientifically valid reasons.

ILLNESSES "LINKED TO HIV"

- **HIV ENCEPHALOPATHY**

Starting with depression, this disorder gradually leads to mental, behavioral, and motor problems. The patient is forgetful, has difficulty in focusing attention, and his reasoning slows down. He loses interest in everything around him and seeks to isolate himself. He is often anxious and irritable. His lower limbs become weak, his steps hesitant and his balance precarious.

The major risk is that this condition may lead to a dement state with severe intellectual impairment, inability to communicate, motor disability and incontinence. Death generally follows within a few months.

When all known causes of encephalitis have been eliminated, the disease is regarded, by default, as HIV related. In fact, the process by which a retrovirus would supposedly act on the brain remains totally unknown, and no explanation has ever been given that could possibly link this type of encephalopathy with immune deficiency.

On another hand, however, certain forms of madness are triggered by intense emotional stress. For example, when a person is declared HIV-positive or, worse still, told that he has AIDS, an illness synonymous with death and rejection by society, dramatic mental havoc frequently occurs. The patient voluntarily isolates himself, and completely loses self-esteem, engendering suicidal thoughts.

HIV CAUSES NUMEROUS ILLNESSES

If the frequently unbearable side effects of antiviral treatments are added to this, it becomes easy to understand why the patient will inexorably sink into severe mental problems, perhaps in desperate attempts to escape horrifying realities or perspectives.

- **HIV ENTEROPATHY**

This chronic diarrhea, usually accompanied by weight loss, and for which no identifiable microbial agent can be found is, again by default, regarded as "HIV" related. Here again, a scientifically demonstrable link is missing.

In fact, this enteropathy is one of the direct consequences of the antiviral therapies that cause, among other side effects, a depletion of the intestinal bacterial flora (we have previously stressed the devastating effects of anti-proteases on digestive functions).

- **WASTING SYNDROME LINKED TO HIV**

Wasting syndrome is characterized by weight loss of more than 10%, accompanied by either persistent diarrhea, fever or chronic weakness, lasting thirty days or more (See the "Bangui" definition of AIDS in chapter 5).

Three types of factors are responsible:

- Psychological and economic factors (fatigue, rejection, social isolation, pain, fear of death, financial distress …);
- Opportunist infections affecting the mouth (oral candidiasis, ulcers…) or the digestive tract (bacterial, fungal or viral infections).
- And, above all, side effects of antiviral drugs, causing diarrhea, nausea, digestive disorders, loss of appetite and taste.

The wasting syndrome was added to the list of AIDS indicator diseases in 1987 because it affected a large number of patients. Its occurrence was attributed to the effects of the retrovirus infection, without ever explaining how. It helped, most unfortunately, to conceal certain devastating effects of the antiviral treatments.

OTHER ILLNESSES

Other, non-infectious illnesses are found which don't come under any of the previous categories. This does not mean that they are HIV linked, but simply that they are found in certain patients during the course of their disease. They include:

- Blood diseases (anemia, septicemia, thrombocytopenia, neutropenia, lactic acidosis.);
- Neurological symptoms (peripheral neuropathies, demyelinating neuropathies, lymphocytic meningitis, vacuolar myelopathy, sensitive polyneuritis, Guillain-Barré syndrome…);
- Various manifestations (such as generalized persistent lymphadenopathy).

In closing, it should be stressed that classic retroviruses such as the Rous sarcoma or the murine leukemia viruses, well known in experimental pathology, never kill the cells they apparently infect. These retroviruses are not, to use the scientific term, "cytolytic". There is therefore no reason to accept the notion that infection by a hypothetical retrovirus could be responsible for some destruction ("lysis") of many circulating CD4 T-lymphocytes, low CD4 counts being part of the definition of AIDS. Low CD4 counts in the circulating blood do not imply that these lymphocytes have been destroyed ("lyzed"). These cells, most likely, have temporarily relocated themselves in connective tissues.

Moreover, in general human pathology, not one single disease has ever been shown to be caused by a retrovirus (See De Harven 1998, under References).

LIE #8
IT'S BETTER TO KNOW THAT YOU ARE HIV-POSITIVE

The catastrophically alarmist prognosis constructed by the sorcerers' apprentices of virology, the media and the health professionals results, for anybody declared HIV-positive, having to face the following equation:

HIV POSITIVITY = AIDS = DEATH.

This (false) dramatic formula has an identical effect on the individual to that used in the practice of witchcraft. Whether one believes in it or not, witchcraft is scaring, its effectiveness being due to the fact that the victim is forewarned of what has been launched at him.

The sorcerer, considered in traditional societies as a holder of esoteric knowledge and magic powers, doesn't have to do anything evil in order to effectively carry out his sinister work. His victim is so convinced that there is nothing he can do to avoid the inevitable result of the witchcraft he is exposed to, that all resistance is futile in face of the occult forces set in motion, and that he will waste away daily until he dies. What leads to this inevitable outcome is intense and prolonged stress, caused not only by the direct action of the sorcerer but also by social isolation, nobody wanting to have anything to do with the cursed individual for fear of reprisals, or from simple superstition.

Nowadays, doctors can act like sort of witchdoctors when they tell one of their patients that they are victims of a fatal and incurable illness, particularly in cases of cancer, but even more surely in cases of AIDS. The propaganda which established the previously quoted equation does the sorcerer's work.

Whereas one often avoids telling a cancer patient about their condition, or uses the utmost care in giving him the bad news, the announcement of HIV positivity (which is not in itself an illness) is frequently done in an abrupt manner, aggravated by alarmist remarks.

Why?

The practitioners hide behind a humanitarian pretext: it is absolutely essential that the patient understands the gravity of his condition so that he immediately accepts antiretroviral therapies which should, in principle, slow down the progress of the infection. The practitioners also try to impose on their patients a sexual hygiene designed to limit the risk of contaminating their partners.

The result of this "bad news policy" is that many people who are in good health but were found "seropositive" swallow dozens of tablets each day, which will progressively weaken their immune system and cause disorders which will be attributed to the virus, further increasing the effects of the medical witchcraft.

STRESS AND AIDS

Acute stress can sometimes have beneficial effects, because it allows the subject to react promptly in the face of an immediate danger (flee or fight). On the other hand, prolonged, chronic stress causes a stream of severe, harmful effects.

Psychological disturbances caused by the pronouncement of HIV-positivity, and the inevitable emotional reactions that follow it, induce physiological reactions which are damaging to

IT'S BETTER TO KNOW THAT YOU ARE HIV-POSITIVE

health by weakening the natural defenses of the body.

More precisely, activation of suprarenal glands and of certain endocrine glands of the brain (hypophysis, hypothalamus, epiphysis) in cases of intense stress, shall inevitably result in the overproduction of certain most important neurotransmitters and chemical messengers like corticosteroids, which are immunosuppressive hormones.

Stress weakens the efficiency of the immune system, but it also provokes numerous other disorders, physical (skin complaints like eczema or psoriasis, respiratory and digestive troubles, alteration in the blood cell counts, increased heart rhythm and raising of arterial pressure...) and psychological (despondency, anxiety, insomnia, excessive anger, fatigue, sadness, disgust with everything, tendency to alcoholism or to drug-addiction...).

In the majority of cases, the psychological stress starts before the screening test. In fact, if someone takes the step of being tested, it is because he believes that he might have done something to put himself "at risk". The obsessive fear of being diagnosed HIV-positive is actually present as soon as the subject decides to check on his serological status.

Once HIV positivity is confirmed, the individual often aggravates his stress, either by voluntary isolation, or as a result of being rejected by his social environment. This last phenomenon is happily less common today than it was in the past, when the psychotic fear of contamination had reached levels bordering on paranoia.

Numerous studies carried out over many years have shown that severe and chronic psychological stress induces symptoms resembling some of those found in AIDS, notably the lowering of the number of CD4-T cells, and the occurrence of illnesses such as pneumonia, tuberculosis, wasting syndrome and dementia (with brain disorders identical to those seen in cases of so-called "dementia linked to HIV").

In addition, the production of corticosteroid hormones is subject to a daily (circadian) cycle whereby the highest blood levels of this hormone are observed early in the morning i.e. at the time when medical laboratories most frequently carry out their tests. Because these hormones cause numerous lymphocytes to rapidly escape from the blood circulation, counts of these cells will probably be lower than if the test had been done in the afternoon or evening.

STRESS AND ANTIVIRALS

As we have seen in chapter 4, anti-retrovirals (ARVs) are dangerous cell poisons provoking numerous, incapacitating side effects.

To expose symptomatic AIDS patients to ARVs is questionable enough. But to prescribe them to people in good health, under the pretext that antibodies have been found in their blood with non-specific tests, is totally inappropriate, and frankly unacceptable from an ethical point of view.

Most incredibly, the blame for the damages caused by these medicines is automatically put on the hypothetical retrovirus. This convinces the patient that the horrible "HIV" is winning the fight, which further weakens his morale and makes him give up hope. To delay the end, he clings with desperation (all that is left to him) to those pills which are doing him so much harm, but which he has been told are his only choice.

Such stress is by its very nature going to precipitate the inevitable, frequently fatal outcome.

The fact that the serological tests lack any real specificity greatly adds to the responsibility of those who prescribe highly toxic medicines to people in good health.

But can an HIV positive individual be considered as in perfect health?

Maybe not. He is currently not ill, but there must be something in his medical history to explain the observed raised level of antibodies.

How should medical practitioners respond in the face of a positive HIV serological test? The first step should unquestionably be to carefully investigate the medical history of the patient. Had he had any blood transfusions, hepatitis, recent vaccinations? Indeed, almost seventy medical conditions are known to frequently result in "seropositivity", and most of those seventy medical conditions have nothing to do with AIDS!

IT'S BETTER TO KNOW THAT YOU ARE HIV-POSITIVE

The worst response, while facing an HIV positive test, is to interpret it as proof of "HIV" infection. Even the pharmaceutical firms' brochures included with the *Elisa* type tests clearly state that a positive reaction couldn't be used in itself as a diagnosis of AIDS. Very sadly, thousands of people have believed, and still do believe in that catastrophic interpretation of the test, and lay themselves open to a torrent of emotional stress, and to serious medicinal poisoning as described above.

All over the world there are hundreds of thousands of healthy "seropositive" individuals, whose health is kept stable by good personal hygiene and a balanced diet, and who do not expose themselves to any antiviral "therapy".

LIE #9
THE AIDS EPIDEMIC IS OVERWHELMING

All public health organizations agree with each other to deliver apocalyptic information on the progress of AIDS throughout the world. This is slavishly relayed (without verification) by the media and all the organizations for which AIDS is their *raison d'être*.

AIDS terror escalates in successive stages:

1. Attributing acquired immunodeficiency to a virus is the first decisive step, creating the idea that AIDS is an infectious transmissible illness.
2. Next is the development of tests for seropositivity, used "officially..." for detecting hypothetical infections in a population in good health (and at the same time inventing heterosexual AIDS).
3. Thirdly, the number of AIDS indicator diseases has been increased, going from three to thirty in a few years.
4. Even the definition of AIDS itself has been significantly modified four times (1982, 1987, 1992 and 1998) by the CDC (Centers for disease control and prevention) and

the WHO (World Health Organization), each new definition resulting in a catastrophic escalation in the apparent epidemic.

5. Finally, acrobatic extrapolations of statistics have increased HIV prevalence each year, above all in countries where appropriate serological, complete verifications are practically impossible to carry out.

Was this "epidemic" situation based on verifiable data?

As early as 1993-1995, Prof. Gordon T. Stewart from Edinburgh, an epidemiologist of considerable experience and authority and who was one of the founding members of the "Rethinking Aids" Group in 1991, had started to raise basic questions on the alleged AIDS "Epidemic". The reader should review his *Lancet* 1993 paper on "Errors in prediction of the incidence and distribution of AIDS", and his *Genetica* 1995 paper on "The Epidemiology and Transmission of AIDS: a hypothesis linking behavioural and biological determinants with time, person and place" (See G. Stewart under References). In spite of these historic warnings, the concept of a "devastating" AIDS epidemic continued to grow, for the highest profit of the pharmaceutical ARV business. Stewart's views and predictions were fully confirmed recently (2007) by James Chin, formerly Chief of the Global Programme on AIDS of the WHO, Geneva, in his book on " The AIDS Pandemic - The Collision of epidemiology with political correctness" (See under References).

What value can be attributed to worldwide statistics, taking into consideration that, in the two regions of the world where AIDS first appeared, the United States and Western Europe, the alleged epidemic has failed to materialize, while in Oceania it hasn't even begun. By contrast, official statistics claim an explosion of HIV prevalence in several geographical areas that had so far been spared.

THE AIDS EPIDEMIC IS OVERWHELMING

THE WORLDWIDE STATISTICS

Reading the annual report of UNAIDS (the official United Nations organization charged with producing worldwide statistics on AIDS) raises indeed serious questions on the reliability of official statistics.

Analysis of the AIDS epidemic – December 2004 is a weighty volume of 95 pages, giving worldwide estimates for the year 2004, as at 1st January 2005.

The following three tables summarize the situation in the main geographical areas around the world, for HIV prevalence, the number of AIDS related deaths, and the number of new infections during the course of the same year, 2004.

Geographical zone	Average estimate	Low estimate	High estimate	Approximation
Sub-Saharan Africa	25,400,000	23,400,000	28,400,000	20%
South and South-East Asia	7,100,000	4,400,000	10,600,000	87%
Latin America	1,700,000	1,300,000	2,200,000	53%
Western Europe and Central Asia	1,400,000	920,000	2,100,000	84%
East Asia	1,100,000	560,000	1,800,000	113%
Caribbean	1,000,000	540,000	1,600,000	106%
North Africa and Middle East	610,000	480,000	760,000	46%
North America	540,000	230,000	1,500,000	235%
Western Europe	440,000	270,000	780,000	116%
Oceania	35,000	25,000	48,000	66%
Total worldwide	39,400,000	35,900,000	44,300,000	22%

Table 4: Official estimates of "infected" people throughout the world as at 1st January 2005 (page 77 of the report)

TEN LIES ABOUT AIDS

Geographical zone	Average estimate	Low estimate	High estimate	Approximation
Sub-Saharan Africa	2,300,000	2,100,000	2,600,000	22%
South and South-East Asia	490,000	300,000	750,000	92%
Latin America	95,000	73,000	120,000	49%
Western Europe and Central Asia	60,000	39,000	87,000	80%
East Asia	51,000	25,000	86,000	120%
Caribbean	36,000	24,000	61,000	103%
North Africa and Middle East	28,000	12,000	72,000	214%
North America	16,000	8,400	25,000	104%
Western Europe	6,500	-	< 8,500	?
Oceania	700	-	< 1,700	?
Total worldwide	3,100,000	2,800,000	3,500,000	23%

Table 5: *Official estimates of deaths due to AIDS during 2004 (page 77 of the report)*

Geographical zone	Average estimate	Low estimate	High estimate	Approximation
Sub-Saharan Africa	3,100,000	2,700,000	3,800,000	35%
South and South-East Asia	890,000	480,000	2,000,000	171%
Latin America	240,000	170,000	430,000	108%
Western Europe and Central Asia	210,000	110,000	480,000	176%
East Asia	290,000	84,000	830,000	257%
Caribbean	53,000	27,000	140,000	213%
North Africa and Middle East	92,000	34,000	350,000	343%
North America	44,000	16,000	120,000	236%
Western Europe	21,000	14,000	38,000	114%
Oceania	5,000	2,100	13,000	218%
Total worldwide	4,900,000	4,300,000	6,400,000	43%

Table 6: *Official estimates newly "infected" people throughout the world during 2004 (page 78 of the report)*

THE AIDS EPIDEMIC IS OVERWHELMING

Table 6 is particularly illustrative of the incoherence of official statistics. It shows estimates of the number of people who have been "infected by HIV" in 2004. How could one explain that the region with the highest level of supervision and control of public health in the world, North America, shows an approximation of 236%? Although less outrageously, the same question applies to Western Europe, with figures of approximately 114%.

Did the investigators have a hard time hacking their way through the jungles of Alsace, or the Bavarian mangroves, to reach the native villages? Of course not!

These estimates were not produced by direct field investigations. Nobody actually went to these places where there was probably not much to see anyway! Statisticians carried out the work by means of computer modeling programs tailor-made to create fear, attract subsidies, and put enormous numbers of people onto medication (See Rian Malan, under References).

The current modeling program is the fourth of its kind, the previous three having been abandoned one by one, because the results they produced were barely credible and could have, eventually, risked questions from political leaders.

A good example is the situation that developed in India a few years ago. The UNAIDS forecasts for that country were very alarmist, predicting 310,000 deaths in 1999. But, the following year, NACO (a non-governmental Indian organization), shocked by the enormity of the forecast figures, carried out its own health survey that showed that between 1986 (the official start of the "epidemic" in India) and 2000, only 1,759 deaths could actually be regarded as AIDS-related.

Alerted by this, the Indian Minister for Health launched a huge screening campaign in Manipur province (supposedly the worst affected), which revealed a seropositivity prevalence rate of 0.4%, as opposed to the 18% previously claimed by the "experts". In the same trend, and as stressed recently in *Science,* July 13, 2007, the official number of people in India supposedly "infected with HIV" was slashed from 5.7 million to 2.5 million.

If political leaders knew that the seropositivity tests, used for "sentinelle" spot checkings, were themselves scientifically unacceptable, perhaps they would have stopped listening to the remote control alarm sirens sounded by the WHO, with the full support of the pharmaceutical industry.

Does it mean that the statistical models used today are more reliable?

No. They are simply craftier. The explanation of the enormous gap between high and low estimates is the so-called "umbrella opening" technique. Also, having seen that increased seropositivity matched the expanding "recreational" drug market in many countries statisticians were able to adjust their numbers by simply referring to police and customs reports showing the extensions of the drug business.

Finally, we must emphasize that UNAIDS experts supplied figures for sub-Saharan AIDS related fatalities with an approximation of (only!) 35%. We are expected to believe that, in these least-medicalized and most difficult to access regions of the world, fatality estimates are seven times more precise than those for the United States. Find the mistake!

AIDS AND WOMEN

During the 80s, AIDS primarily affected male homosexuals living in the big cities (61% of cases in the USA), drug addicts of both sexes (21%), and a minority of people who had had blood transfusions (2%). Seven percent of patients were both homosexuals and drug addicts. The new plague primarily affected men belonging to high risk groups (which is still the case today, despite what we are told, but in agreement with James Chin's recent report).

This was so obvious that, as already indicated, the first name for AIDS was "GRID" (*Gay Related Immune Deficiency* - Immune deficiency in homosexuals*).*

From 1986 onwards, a huge campaign was designed to strike fear into the hearts of heterosexuals, as we saw in the previous chapter. Ever since, everybody has believed that AIDS can affect women just as well as men, non-drug abusers as much as addicts, heterosexuals as well as homosexuals. Seropositivity antibody tests have done a great deal to consolidate this nonsense.

THE AIDS EPIDEMIC IS OVERWHELMING

Going back to UNAIDS reports, which devote a whole chapter to women, and analyzing **table 7**, we find that women reportedly represent 25% of infected adults in western countries (North America and Western Europe), while this percentage increases to 57% in sub-Saharan Africa.
Could it be that HIV preferably infects black women?

Geographical zone	Percentage of women
Sub-Saharan Africa	57%
South and South-East Asia	30%
Latin America	36%
Western Europe and Central Asia	34%
East Asia	22%
Caribbean	49%
North Africa and Middle East	48%
North America	25%
Western Europe	25%
Oceania	21%
Average worldwide	47%

Table 7: Percentage of women among adults supposedly infected at 1st January 2005 (page 5 of the report)

Rather than making presumptions with unacceptable racist overtones, health authorities prefer to hide behind the hypothesis that, in Africa and in other areas like the Caribbean, North Africa and the Middle East, contamination mostly occurs via the heterosexually route. This explanation of African women's contamination is also the result of racial prejudices that claim that most Africans lead an unbridled, even depraved sex life, which is totally untrue. Remember, moreover, that sexual transmission of HIV has never been satisfactorily documented, since nobody has ever seen HIV particles directly in the blood or in the sperm of any AIDS patient...

Informative comments are as follows (translation according to a document in French):

Page 8, we can see that, in India:

> " ... near 90% of seropositive women received in prenatal consultations affirm they have only had a single long term relation" (Cohen – 2004).

Apparently, faithful married seropositive women have been infected by their spouse, who has himself been infected during extra-marital sexual intercourse (without any real evidence, since the seropositivity of the incriminated husbands was never verified).

Page 9:

> "Afro-American and Hispanic women represent less than a quarter of the total feminine gender in United States but, in 2000, they account for 80% of the AIDS cases notified among women" (CDC – 2002).

Statistically, AIDS in the USA develops mostly in women from the most deprived groups. How can this phenomenon be explained, if not by the fact that it is also among these groups that the largest contingent of drug addicts and persons are found, among individuals living in extreme poverty?

Page 10:

> "Among a population of young women between 15 and 19 in Kisumu – Kenya and Ndola – Zambia, a multicenter study reveled that the HIV infection levels was 10% higher for married women than for sexually active single women" (Glynn et al – 2001).
>
> "In rural areas of Uganda, among women between 15 and 19 infected by HIV, 88% of them were married" (Kelly et al – 2003). "The reason is the fact that young women, and particularly the teenagers) are married with men more aged, these men having a large probability to have had others sexual partners and, therefore, to have been exposed to HIV".

THE AIDS EPIDEMIC IS OVERWHELMING

Therefore, it appears more dangerous for women in these countries to be married, than single and sexually liberated! As for the increased risk of infection according to the age of the spouse, it is the age group of 25-35 that has always paid the heaviest tribute to AIDS.
Page 12:

> " *Research reveled strong links between violence of life partner and an increased probability of HIV infection" (Heise, Ellsberg and Gottemoeller – 1999).*
>
> " *A study performed in Kigali – Rwanda among women with stable relation has showed that HIV-positive women had higher probabilities to have had a past history of physical and sexual violence due to their male partner than HIV-negative women" (Van der Straten et al – 1998).*

The following quotation explains what WHO means by "violence against women":

> " *Violence against women means various types of behavior, particularly sexual violence (rape or forced sexual relation), sexual aggression, psychological cruelty (for example, to prevent a woman to see her family or friends), defamation, continual humiliation or intimidation and economical restrictions (for example, to prevent a woman to have a job or to confiscate her pay)".*

Women living in highly precarious conditions are more likely to react positively to the serological test. What more do we need to understand that the tests in question indicate the presence of antibodies developed by people in a situation of physical distress, and not in response to an hypothetical "HIV" contamination?
Page 12 (education and HIV):

> " *... But the relationship between education and HIV is complex.*
> *In Burkina Faso, HIV level among pregnant women was the higher for women with a primary school degree or who have not finished their secondary cycle (2.9 and 2.6 % respectively).*

TEN LIES ABOUT AIDS

> *The lower prevalence was found among women who had finished their secondary cycle (1.6 %) or who had never gone at school (1.9 %)" (Ministry of health, Burkina Faso – 2003).*
>
> *" In Ghana, HIV prevalence among pregnant women with a primary education was near two times higher (2.8 %) than among women who had never gone to school (1.5 %) and a third party higher (2.1 %) than women who had finished their secondary cycle" (Ghana statistical service and al. – 2003).*
>
> *" In addition, the last surveillance cycle in Nigeria has shown that infection levels was higher among pregnant women with a primary school degree (5.6 %) and lower among women with high school degree and those who had never received any education at school (4 % and 3.8 % respectively)" (Federal Ministry of health, Nigeria – 2003).*
>
> *" The link between lack of education and low HIV level could be relative to geographic factors or others".*

Oh, what beautiful statistics!

Apparently, women who have never been to school have the lowest rate of seropositivity. And "experts" don't understand why! Could it be that the virus preferably attacks the uneducated?

It would be better to admit that this type of statistical study is insignificant, since it refers to the criterion of education, which has nothing to do with the viral infectiousness.

On the other hand, one could imagine that women not having had access to school make up part of the groups living far from the big towns, therefore often from peasant families, and possibly better fed than the average citizen. This nutritional factor could possibly explain why highly educated women, i.e. from wealthy families (everything being relative), have quite similar results to those of uneducated women.

Note that all the statistical studies quoted by the UNAIDS report were carried out on pregnant women, apparently disregarding the fact that, as previously stressed, pregnancy itself is a documented cause of false positives.

Page 14:

> *" Microbicides (germ-killers) promise a prevention tool controlled by women. The simulation shows that a microbicide,*

THE AIDS EPIDEMIC IS OVERWHELMING

even at only 60 % effective, could have an important result if it will be introduced in the 73 countries of the world where revenue is lower. If such a product was used by only 20 % of women already in relation with health services, it could prevent 2.5 millions new infections among women, men and infants, by three years".

" ... Nowadays, the private market don't bring fund enough for microbicides, despite the fact that appraisals argue a 1.8 billion dollars market by 2020 for an effective product" (Access Working Group – 2000).

Are microbicides an attractive future market? The reason why pharmaceutical companies are not yet leaping into this promising area is perhaps because marketing of anti-retrovirals is still far more lucrative, at least for a few more years. A question open for future investigation is whether or not microbicides might also act as spermicides, possibly interfering with fertilization and birth control, without the treated individuals being aware?

AFRICAN AIDS

Reporting from African countries where AIDS is reportedly rampant, the media never stop over-emphasizing decimated villages and starving orphans wandering along the roads.

An English journalist from the Sunday Times, Neville Hodgkinson, put things into perspective as early as 1993, while on a trip to Central Africa ("the epicenter" of the epidemic, at the time) in order to witness the horror of the situation. He was very surprised by what he found.

People told him that the inhabitants of these deserted villages weren't dead, but had migrated to the cities where they hoped to find food to alleviate their hunger. The improvised bush cemeteries where virus victims were reportedly hurriedly buried for fear of contagion (as widely mentioned in the Western press) were probably invented by media reporters, responding to a never-ending demand for horror and sensationalism.

As a Ghanaian doctor, Dr Félix Konotey-Ahulu, rightly remarked: "Since Africans don't practice cremation, if AIDS is killing so many victims, where are the graves?"

South African journalist Rian Malan published a most important appraisal of the African AIDS situation in London's *The Spectator* in December 2003, and later in France in the *Courrier International* in February 2004.

Reacting to a press coverage shown to him by one of his friends, stating that Botswana was so decimated by AIDS that its population had gone from 1.4 million to less than one million people in ten years, and that the country would soon disappear from the map, Rian Malan presented the following official demographic data:

> *"Botswana has just concluded a census that shows population growing at about 2.7 per cent a year, in spite of what is usually described as the worst Aids problem on the planet. Total population has risen to 1.7 million in just a decade. If anything, Botswana is experiencing a minor population explosion.*
>
> *There is similar bad news for the doomsayers in Tanzania's new census, which shows population growing at 2.9 per cent a year. Professional pessimists will be particularly discomforted by developments in the swamplands west of Lake Victoria, where HIV first emerged, and where the depopulated villages of popular mythology are supposedly located. Here, in the district of Kagera, population grew at 2.7 per cent a year before 1988, only to accelerate to 3.1 per cent even as the Aids epidemic was supposedly peaking. Uganda's latest census tells a broadly similar story, as does South Africa's.*
>
> *Some might think it good news that the impact of Aids is less devastating than most laymen imagine, but they are wrong. In Africa, the only good news about Aids is bad news, and anyone who tells you otherwise is branded a moral leper, bent on sowing confusion and derailing 100,000 worthy fundraising drives."*

Charles Geshekter, Professor of African History at the California State University in Chico, California, having made numerous site visits to different African countries, pointed his finger at many official inconsistencies in an article published in March 2000 in the Toronto *Globe and Mail* newspaper (extracts):

THE AIDS EPIDEMIC IS OVERWHELMING

"The most reliable statistics on AIDS in Africa are found in the WHO's Weekly Epidemiological Record. The total cumulative number of AIDS cases reported in Africa since 1982, when AIDS record-keeping began, is 794,444 -- a number starkly at odds with the latest scare figures, which claim 2.3 million AIDS deaths throughout Africa for 1999 alone."

Later, he recounts one of the experiences he had during his last visit to the Republic of South Africa:

"Beauty Nongila, principal of a rural school in north Zululand, insisted that having more toilets would improve the health of her 408 students (her sparsely-equipped elementary school has four). She struggled to provide her underfed kids with a spartan lunch on an allowance of 8 cents a day. When I inquired about the AIDS crisis, she laughed and said that dental problems, respiratory illnesses, diarrhea and chronic hunger were far more vexing."

Obviously, AIDS spreads in Africa differently from the way it does in developed countries, women being considerably more affected.

Why this difference? Officially, it is because of the high frequency of heterosexual contamination! What haven't we heard about the sexual habits of African men? Sexual activity starting at puberty; sodomy practiced as a means of contraception; sex with monkeys; continual changing of partners; insatiable sexual appetite...

How can people make such unacceptably racist remarks?

In another article published in October 1994 in the *New African* magazine, Charles Geshekter explains:

"In fact, there is little evidence to support Western perceptions of African sexual promiscuity. Widespread modesty codes for women, whose sexuality is considered a gift to be used for procreation, make many African societies seem chaste compared to the West. The Somalis, Afars, Oromos and Amharas of northeast Africa think that public displays of sexual feelings demean a woman's "gift," so that sexual contacts are restricted to ceremonial touching or dancing. Initial sexual relationships

TEN LIES ABOUT AIDS

> *are geared to the beginnings of making a family. The notion of "boyfriends" and "girlfriends," virtually universal in the West, has no parallel in most traditional African cultures."*

There's a huge gap between the statistical models repeatedly presented by the epidemiologists and the actual truth. While estimates of the sexually active African population are 3.5 partners per year, studies on the ground show to the contrary, that sexuality in Africa is the same as in other regions of the world, and even less than in some western countries.

For example, a study carried out in twelve African countries in 1995 showed that 74% of men and 91% of women in the age group 15-49 had only had sex with their usual partner during the previous year. These figures are comparable to those shown in similar studies carried out, at the same time, in Denmark, Great Britain and France.

The sexual promiscuity of Africans is also a myth. A joint study carried out in 1991 by *Médecins Sans Frontières* and the *Harvard School of Public Health* in the Moyo district (north-west of Uganda) showed that the average age of the first sexual intercourse was seventeen years for women and nineteen years for men. Sex before marriage was only found in 18% of women and 50% of men. As for sexual infidelity, it only affected 2% of women and 15% of men during the year prior to the study.

THE AIDS ORPHANS

As Charles Geshekter rightly pointed out in the previously quoted article, the figures regarding children orphaned by AIDS also need to be critically reappraised. Three parameters have to be taken into account: the average rate of fertility in African women, which is 5.8; the very high infant mortality; and the average life span of Africans (fifty for women and forty-seven for men).

> *" ... so it would not be surprising, on a continent of 650 million people, if there were not even more than 10 million children whose mothers had died before they reached high-school age."*

THE AIDS EPIDEMIC IS OVERWHELMING

The Austrian obstetrician, Dr Christian Fiala, having made several humanitarian/medical missions to Africa, puts this into perspective (private communications to the authors, and see under References):

> " In Uganda, the definition of orphan is not the same than in Europe. An infant is declared orphan if he/she doesn't live with both mother and father. Attention: this doesn't signify that one or other parent is death but only that the family structure is only composed of the father or the mother. While it is known that the greater part of Ugandan's women have children from different fathers, it is easy to understand that many of these infants are considered as orphans.
>
> If this Ugandan definition was applied in Europe, there immediately would be millions of orphans because there are numerous separate couples".

AN EXAMPLE IN TANZANIA

Among the numerous humanitarian groups working in Africa, some are independent from the heavily publicized and subsidized programs. This is the case of *"Partage Tanzanie"*, an association lead by a former pilot who became a health officer and the leader of a vast humanitarian program, Philippe Krynen.

This NGO looks after Tanzanian orphans in the north-west of Tanzania, watered by the Kagera river, an area considered at the beginning of the 90s as one most affected by AIDS.

How did that happen in this enclave between Rwanda and Uganda, bordered on the east by Lake Victoria?

Marc Deru, a Belgian physician who spent several months working with Philippe Krynen, explains:

> " This area was, at the beginning of 20th century, considered like a little paradise: climate is favorable (altitude: 1200 meters) with mild rains throughout the year; around each house, banana trees give, as well as beans growing under their foliage, a luxuriant basic foods; products of fishing complete this feeding; the coffee market development

bring cash to inhabitants; infants go to school, on place or in Uganda for secondary cycle.

But, since the second world war, a crop of events bring about a complete turnaround of this idyllic situation: a disease, the West Coast fever, exterminate the bovine livestock. Banana trees decline (by lack of their natural enriching agent, the cow pat) and after several decades are victim of a fungus disease.

In addition, the offering price of coffee breaks down, nationalizations (from 1967) demolish the sanitary and academic networks and, ultimate disaster, in 1979, the war conducted by Idi Amin Dada against Tanzania devastates the region.

Malnutrition takes hold durably. Basic products lack. Infants who survive become immune afflicted adults and mortality by TB, other respiratory diseases, intestinal infection and massive parasitism, added to chronic malaria, is very important. A calamitous sanitary and farming situation pushes the survivors to expatriate and try one's luck in the great towns of Eastern Africa".

At the beginning of the 80s, the Kagera region was an area devastated by rampant endemic illnesses and famine, both causing severe immunodeficiency.

When Philippe Krynen and his wife visited the north of Tanzania for the first time in 1988, they found an apocalyptic situation, and decided to organize a health rescue program for the innumerable destitute and abandoned children in this region.

The following year, *"Partage Tanzanie"* started a program of development and care, covering thirty villages. Philippe Krynen noticed as time went on:

- the children, whether seropositive or seronegative, equally recovered when they were properly fed and treated;
- the tests showing positive results when they were done during an infection, were negative a few months later;
- systematic screening of all the inhabitants of a village (842 people) revealed a seropositivity rate of 13.8%, while the WHO announced HIV prevalence of 40% to 50% in that region.

THE AIDS EPIDEMIC IS OVERWHELMING

He consequently publicly reported on his doubts as to the viral origin of AIDS. This resulted in him being considered a dangerous "dissident" by those who had previously been so supportive to him as long as he shared the official alarmist attitude about the extent of the so-called "epidemic".

The support which he had been promised by the European Union never materialized, and "*Partage Tanzanie*" owes its current survival and remarkable success to the generosity and commitment of many private philanthropists.

The results obtained by this small independent NGO are exceptional, with a spectacular fall in the infant mortality rate, which is now only one quarter of the regional rate.

Appropriate and balanced diet, clean drinking water, adequate sanitation, the use of mosquito nets, specific treatment of ailments, but also a great deal of love and affection have succeeded in overcoming chronic immunodeficiency in this area, without any ARV medication. There is no distribution of condoms, and useless so-called HIV antibody tests are never carried out.

The Tanzanian government having for its part created an effective health and social campaign, the whole region is coming back to life, distancing itself from the threat of a virtual epidemic.

OTHER REGIONS OF THE WORLD

Reading the entire UNAIDS report raises considerable ambiguity, mostly because it perpetuates the complete confusion between seropositivity, supposedly "people living with HIV", and patients actually "suffering from AIDS".

Anybody reading the report will therefore be given to believe that the reported figures concern individuals who are victims of illnesses linked to AIDS, while this has never been demonstrated.

On the other hand, the studies of risk factors only mention intravenous drug users, which falsifies the data. The viral hypothesis assumes that infection is uniquely through the blood, and blames the syringes. In reality, and as known for many years prior to the advent of AIDS, all hard drugs cause immunodeficiency to a greater or lesser degree, and are directly responsible for different health problems. No mention is made of cocaine (more widespread, however), inhaled drugs (poppers, crack), nor other narcotics that are almost as harmful.

Countries in the inter-tropical zone suffer not only from poverty but also from many endemic illnesses, which falsify statistics, many of these infections having symptoms listed as being signs of AIDS.

The majority of cases of lowered immunity in certain Caribbean islands (notably Haiti), in Asia, Central America and South America can primarily be explained by malnutrition.

The UNAIDS report stresses sexual behavior, whether homosexual or heterosexual. Prostitution is indicated as being a major factor in the transmission of the illness. But, as we have already emphasized, prostitutes show an extremely low (almost nil) incidence of AIDS, throughout the world, seropositivity being reported only among prostitutes who are also IV drug abusers. The extremely low incidence of HIV/AIDS among prostitutes is in total conflict with James Chin's conclusions, namely that AIDS occurs only among high risk subjects exposing themselves to very promiscuous, multiple partners sexual behavior.

Actually, statistics of the said "HIV infection" parallel impressively those of drug abuse that affects more and more regions of the world, as emphasized in the following note coming from the Russian Federation :

> *" It is estimate that between 1.5 and 3 millions Russians shoot drugs (1 to 2% of total population)".*
>
> *" A multicenter study estimated that 65 % of injectable drugs consumers in Irkousk's streets was HIV-positive (of witch 90% are teenagers). In Tver, 55% were infected. In Ekaterinebourg, this number was 34%, and in Samara 29% (Rhodes et al. – 2004).*

Concerning prostitution:

> *" ... Nevertheless, one of the most detailed studies to date was performed in Saint-Petersburg where 81% of prostitutes who*

THE AIDS EPIDEMIC IS OVERWHELMING

participated to this survey declared to use drugs by injection (principally heroin) at least once a day, and among them, 65% had used non-sterile material. Almost all (96%) claimed to use a condom during their last sexual intercourse. However, a screening test revealed that 48% of them were HIV-positive".

Finally, a phenomenon should be mentioned which has particularly affected central China where very poor people sell their blood to private companies. Many of these people have been bled most abusively, giving blood more than once a week over several years. It is no surprise that this totally unethical practice, aggravated by malnutrition, has led to a great number of cases of immune deficiency that, when geographically clustered, made it look like an epidemic.

LIE #10
THE SCIENTISTS ALL AGREE

Everybody thinks that scientists unanimously believe that HIV is the cause of AIDS.

In truth, a considerable majority of members of the medical profession and of the bio-medical research community are sincerely convinced that a virus called "HIV" is the cause of the acquired immunodeficiency syndrome. In spite of the fact that the HIV-AIDS hypothesis was then, and remains un-proven, it was blindly accepted, almost unanimously, by the media, the pharmaceutical companies and the professional publications. The resulting bias has been so dominant over the past 20 years that all attempts to set up alternative research programs have been paralyzed, with no alternative, non-viral hypothesizes having received any serious attention.

Nevertheless, several hundreds of eminent scientists, at the risk of jeopardizing their academic careers, have chosen to focus their attention on toxic, pharmaceutical, behavioral and nutritional possible alternative causes of AIDS.

HISTORY OF THE CONTROVERSY

In 1987, Peter Duesberg, microbiology professor at the University of California at Berkeley, began to seriously question the viral hypothesis of AIDS, in a publication that appeared in *Cancer Research*.

A scientist of considerable international reputation, Duesberg was a leading member of the National Academy of Sciences of the USA and had made classic research contributions in the field of oncogenes (genes implicated in cancers). He was also an uncontested retrovirus expert, from the molecular genetics point of view .

He was first in courageously raising key questions such as:

- How could a dormant and inactive virus kill billions of cells when it only infected a few?
- How could this virus be responsible for a fatal illness when it is almost undetectable, even in patients in the terminal stage?
- Why are there AIDS patients in whom it is impossible to find the least trace of HIV?
- Why have none of the numerous laboratory animals infected ever developed AIDS?

The scientific community totally ignored these embarrassing questions, because they evidently underline the fact that many control experiments were missing in the construct on which the HIV paradigm was based. From that time on, silence has always been the most convenient escape to the embarrassment of unanswerable questions about the HIV theory of AIDS.

For firmly maintaining his positions, Peter Duesberg became the target of a systematic academic rejection campaign. He was no longer invited to attend conferences, and scientific journals started refusing to publish his papers. Moreover, his research grant budget was soon drastically cut.

However, courageous and dedicated scientists joined Peter Duesberg in his fight for the truth, and in 1991, under the initiative of Professor Charles Thomas, biochemist at Harvard, founded the "Group for the Scientific Reappraisal of the HIV-AIDS hypothesis". The initial meeting included Peter Duesberg,

THE SCIENTISTS ALL AGREE

Charles Thomas, Gordon Stewart, Harry Rubin, Richard Strohman, Phil Johnson, and Steve Jonas. It is frequently referred to as "The Group", or RA (for Reappraising Aids), and soon started to publish an important newsletter "Rethinking Aids", Paul Philpott serving as a most dedicated editor for over a decade.

"The Group" invited "AIDS dissidents" to sign in support of the following statement:

> *"It is widely believed by the general public that a retrovirus called HIV causes the group of diseases called AIDS. Many biomedical scientists now question this hypothesis. We propose that a thorough reappraisal of the evidence for and against this hypothesis be conducted by a suitable independent group. We further propose that critical epidemiological studies be devised and undertaken."*

Several prominent scientific journals have refused to publish this statement (although it was finally published in *Science* in 1995), a statement that has now been signed by over 2,600 scientists, health professionals and concerned citizens.

Charles Thomas later stated: *"I think that, for a scientist, to remain silent while facing such serious doubts is equivalent to criminal negligence."*

Actually, at that time, many scientists revolted against the authorities and lobbies who dogmatically maintained a viral theory that had so little credibility.

Even Luc Montagnier, the "co-discoverer of HIV", began to modulate his position, provoking the anger of his colleagues by announcing, during a conference in San Francisco in 1990, that the virus could not cause AIDS without the intervention of a "co-factor".

The same applies to John Maddox, editor of the illustrious scientific magazine, *Nature*. In an editorial, he regretted not having had faith in Peter Duesberg's arguments, when numerous studies had shown them to be valid. Maddox's courage was short-lived, since a retraction followed one month later!

The RA "Group", founded in 1991, grew larger and larger. The number of signatories to the declaration of this group kept growing during the 90s. The signatories (now more than 2,600) comprise a great number of scientists of great renown, including two Nobel Prize laureates. Although initially centered in California, the "Group" soon took on an international profile, the signatures of the initial RA statement coming from all over the United States, and very soon from Europe, Australia and the rest of the world. One of the authors of this book (ÉDH) served from 2005 until 2008, as President of RA.

In 1991, a prestigious medical journal, *The Lancet*, published an article seriously questioning the validity of the principal serological test (the *Western Blot* test). The lack of specificity of this test was confirmed in 1993 by a group of Australian researchers, working in Perth, who published their study in another high-level scientific journal, *Nature/Biotechnology*. The Australian group, comprising Eleni Papadopulos, Valendar Turner and several others, lost no time in establishing themselves as eloquent spokesmen for ideas that began to be described as those of the "AIDS dissidents".

Fundamental "dissident" publications, starting with those of Peter Duesberg in 1987, were simply ignored by the "official" research establishment, where it was evident that research on AIDS had shifted one hundred percent into "HIV" research. This shift of emphasis, which raises considerable questions into the integrity of medical science in our countries, soon attracted the attention of several brave journalists. In the United States we should mention Celia Farber, who in 1992 published an historic alarm call, stressing the absence of any scientific credibility in the official hypothesis of "HIV" being the cause of AIDS.

The same year, Neville Hodgkinson in the United Kingdom published his observations made during a long journey in equatorial Africa, raising profound doubts regarding what the daily newspapers described as the catastrophic ravages of AIDS in African populations. He stressed the dominant role played by lack of hygiene, lack of drinking water, and by malnutrition in creating the serious public health problems he observed in the countries he visited.

The reality of an "AIDS epidemic" in America and Europe had initially been very seriously questioned (*Lancet*, 1993), as

THE SCIENTISTS ALL AGREE

already mentioned by Professor Gordon Stewart. The concept of an "epidemic", officially based on the contagiousness of "HIV", was soon rocked even harder in 1994 when a German virologist, Stefan Lanka, voiced the most serious doubts about the very existence of "HIV". Numerous dissidents began, at this time, to ask themselves questions about the scientific validity of the methods used in 1983-1984, methods that had led to the pretended isolation of "HIV". And today, doubts about the very existence of "HIV" are shared by a majority of dissidents!

The diffusion of dissident views was considerably accelerated by the publication, in London, of the magazine *Continuum*, founded by Jody Wells, and to which the editor, the late Huw Christie, has brought major contributions, collaborating with Joan Shenton and several other consultants who are today among the most active members of the international dissident movement. But, despite all these efforts to communicate, open debates between the dissidents and the orthodoxy are still extremely rare events.

In France, however, Djamel Tahi, a Parisian journalist, succeeded in 1996 in presenting an important open debate on the Arte television channel. The very informative contribution of Renaud Russeil, who published (in Switzerland) his book *Enquête sur le sida – Les vérités muselées* (Inquiry into AIDS – the Muzzled Truth) in 1996, must equally be stressed.

Censorship of the general practitioners' press is as rigorous as that of medical journals. Hints as to the very existence of a dissident movement in the French or international press are extremely rare, or otherwise openly sarcastic.

The two authors of this book are well aware of the censorship exercised by the media. The work by Jean-Claude Roussez published in 2004 under the title: *"Sida: supercherie scientifique et arnaque humanitaire"* ("AIDS: Scientific Trickery and Humanitarian Swindles") was sent to the press offices of numerous daily and weekly newspapers, radio and television producers (certain of which owe their reputation to a pretended freedom of expression), unfortunately with no response!

Étienne de Harven, for his part, submitted to *Le Monde* newspaper many reader's letters which, in the most restrained and precise terms, tried to correct certain disinformation relative to AIDS.

Not one of these letters was ever published.

The press being totally unreceptive to "non-HIV" ideas, the Internet remains the best mode of worldwide communication and debate. This has been remarkably exemplified in France by the late Mark Griffiths, who developed the *Sidasanté* website that has made an enormous contribution to public information on AIDS dissidence. Mark Griffiths put years of intense work on the construction of his website (www.sidasante.com) that remains a basic reference for all French-speaking countries. He very suddenly passed away in October 2004. Please note that this book is most affectionately dedicated to his memory.

Dissidents do not have any access to the major international conferences on AIDS. They are automatically excluded. There was, however, an exception in 1998, due to the efforts of Michael Baumgartner who managed to arrange for a large presentation by several dissidents during the 12th World AIDS Conference that was held in Geneva that year.

However, AIDS dissidence took on another dimension in 2000.

That year, the President of the Republic of South Africa, Mr. Thabo Mbeki, wanted to verify the accuracy of the official information available on what was called "AIDS" in sub-Saharan Africa. To that effect, he convened a large international conference on AIDS in Africa, at his government's expense. Thabo Mbeki invited an approximately equal number of orthodox and dissident scientists.

The first conference was held in Pretoria in May 2000. The attending dissidents (all MDs or PhDs) comprised, in alphabetical order: Harvey Bialy, Étienne de Harven, Peter Duesberg, Christian Fiala, Charles Geshekter, Roberto Giraldo, Claus Koehnlein, Manu Kothari, Sam Mhlongo, Eleni Papadopulos, David Rasnik, Gordon Stewart and Valendar Turner. Kary Mullis was also invited, but was unfortunately unable to attend. All of them are therefore part of the Presidential AIDS Advisory Panel.

The objective, of the first conference in Pretoria was to or-

THE SCIENTISTS ALL AGREE

ganize an "orthodox/dissident" working group, with many members who had never previously met.

It was during this first conference that one of the authors of this book (ÉDH) formally pointed out that no "HIV" particles had ever been seen with an electron microscope in the blood of supposedly "high viral load" AIDS patients. This claim has never yet been contradicted. At the end of the conference, a discussion forum was organized regarding the setting up of a new Internet site, with the aim of facilitating exchanges and criticisms between all the members of the panel for a period of two months, and in preparation for the conference second round that took place in Johannesburg in July.

During the second conference, it was unfortunately evident that the positions of the two "camps" had remained totally unchanged.

However, a general consensus was reached on two important points, which were:

1. That, admittedly, the epidemiological data provided by the South African health authorities in the summer of 2000 were quite insufficient to allow the organization of a rational and effective health policy;
2. That a series of ten control experiments should be undertaken, experiments that were deemed essential for the much-needed verification of the HIV/AIDS hypothesis.

The South African government had promised to cover the costs of these ten experiments, whose protocols had been carefully discussed and agreed upon. With one exception, none of these experiments has ever been carried out, not for lack of funds, but mainly because of the difficulty in finding South African laboratories prepared to co-operate with AIDS dissidents!

President Mbeki's efforts remain, however, a turning point for the dissident organization, because for the first time a head of government had given his complete support to a debate on AIDS, a debate in which the key role of "HIV" was clearly brought into question.

How intolerable that was for the orthodoxy that needed to immediately remove this stain! To do so, a group of "181 scientists and front line physicians" immediately wrote a "Letter" which was published in record time in *Nature* (No. 406, 15-16, 2000) and which is known under the name of "The Durban Declaration". This letter contained the most dogmatic assertions and falsehoods, and was supported by several thousand signatures, including those of David Baltimore, Aaron Klug, Luc Montagnier, and a great many others!

A reply to this "Declaration" was quickly published in *Nature* under the title "The Durban Declaration is not accepted by all" (Gordon Stewart et al., *Nature* No. 407 of 21st September 2000) that documents extremely well the title of this chapter "The scientists all agree" as being one of the ten lies analyzed in this book...

Another major debate was held in the Brussels European Parliament, on December 8, 2003. It was organized primarily by the European Deputy Paul Lannoye and by Dr. Marc Deru, under the title "AIDS in Africa". The debate was public, and was followed by long discussions (in which Luc Montagnier actively participated). The proceedings of this symposium were published, in French, in 2004 (see under References). The press had been largely invited to the debate, but rigorous censorship being what it is, not the least reference to this debate appeared in the Brussels newspapers on the following days.

The conclusion of this chapter is evident:

The most official members of the scientific mainstream of AIDS research have had numerous opportunities to hear about the dissident position that completely rejects the hypothetical viral cause of AIDS. It is false to say "The scientists all agree". No, they all choose to ignore dissenting views and consistently avoid exposing themselves to open debates that would be dangerously dominated by "Evidence Based Medicine"! To keep dollars flowing in, and to avoid public embarrassment is the rule among members of the AIDS orthodoxy. Only when invitations for a debate originate from very high levels, such as from President Mbeki, and from the European Parliament, would they possibly sacrifice a few hours from their busy schedules,

THE SCIENTISTS ALL AGREE

making sure, however, never to displease the heads of the big pharmaceutical firms, whose support is essential for the thriving "HIV" business...

In 2001, David Rasnick, member of T. Mbeki AIDS Advisory panel, wrote a striking page on "The Aids Blunder" in the Mail and Guardian, Johannesburg, South Africa, 24th January, that is highly relevant to the main points made in this chapter and shall be quoted here completely, with kind permission of the author.

THE AIDS BLUNDER

The contagious, HIV hypothesis of AIDS is the biggest scientific, medical blunder of the 20th Century. The evidence is overwhelming that AIDS is not contagious, sexually transmitted, or caused by HIV. I have come to realize that embarrassment is the main obstacle to exposing this simple fact.

So why are we barraged, almost daily, by an endless litany of AIDS horrors and HIV statistics? Why do virtually all doctors and public health officials profess their unswerving allegiance to the unproven hypothesis that AIDS is contagious and sexually transmitted when the evidence is greatly against it?

There are more than a hundred thousand doctors and scientists who have built their careers and reputations by simply accepting the articles of faith about AIDS. At this late date, it is simple human embarrassment that is the biggest obstacle to bringing the AIDS insanity to an end. It is the fear of being so obviously and hopelessly wrong about AIDS that keeps lips sealed, the money flowing and AIDS rhetoric spiraling to stratospheric heights of absurdity.

The physicians who know or suspect the truth are embarrassed or afraid to admit that the HIV tests are absurd and should be outlawed, and that the anti-HIV drugs are injuring and killing people. We are taught to fear antibodies, and to believe that antibodies to HIV are a harbinger of disease and death ten years in the future. When you protest this absurdity and point out to health care workers that antibodies are the very essence of antiviral immunity your objections are met with either contempt or embarrassed silence.

TEN LIES ABOUT AIDS

The National Institutes of Health, the Centers for Disease Control, the Medical Research Council of South Africa, and the World Health Organization are terrorizing hundreds of millions of people around the world by their reckless and absurd policy of equating sex with death. Self preservation compels these institutions to not only maintain but to actually compound their errors, which adds to the fear, suffering, and misery of the world - the antithesis of their reason for being.

The only way we can free ourselves from the AIDS blunder and bring an end to the tyranny of fear is to have an open international discourse and debate on all things AIDS. Anger will be a natural response to facing the enormity of the scandal of AIDS. Anger has its place but it should be put aside quickly. It is a mistake to focus on villains and on whom to punish. The AIDS blunder is a sociological phenomenon in which we all share a measure of responsibility.

Ultimately, the AIDS blunder is not really about AIDS, nor even about health and disease, nor even about science and medicine. The AIDS blunder is about the health of our democracies. A healthy democracy demands that its citizens keep a skeptical, even suspicious, eye on its institutions in order to prevent them from becoming the autonomous, authoritarian regimes they are now.

The AIDS blunder shows that we need to rethink and restructure our institutions of government, science, health, academe, journalism and media. We must replace the National Institutes of Health as the primary gatekeeper of research funding with numerous competing sources of funding. We must restructure the peer review processes of scientific publishing and funding so that they do not promote and protect any particular dogma or fashion of thought or exclude competing ideas. A robust and mean investigative journalism must be revived, rewarded and cherished.

Finally, as citizens we must take back the authority and responsibility for our own health and well being and that of our democracies."

ENOUGH LIES

The official hypothesis, which claims that AIDS is caused by a retrovirus, has never been scientifically verified. Economic interests, lobbying pressure groups, and "politically correct" maneuvers, however, gave dogmatic credibility to this hypothesis over the past twenty or more years, against all scientifically available data.

One can only hope that readers of this book will understand the extent of the damage (physical, psychological, societal, etc...) that has been done, worldwide, by the erroneous HIV hypothesis.

The anguish that is created, undeservedly, when a person is declared seropositive, added to the severe side effects of the alleged "antiretroviral therapies", added also to ostracism and exclusion, represent the most frequently encountered facets of the tragedy. How long will it take for the appropriate questions to be openly debated, and the current, scandalous situation to be resolved?

Recent books, written by concerned scientists (see H. Bauer, J. Chin, R. Culshaw, all published in 2007) all point in the same direction, i.e. questioning the current paradigm either from the epidemiological or the virological viewpoint. Can we anticipate that these books shall be received in a more objective, dispassionate way, and consequently bring many health professionals to finally open their eyes?

Most obviously, the cost of medical research has never stopped escalating. Consequently, research directions are inescapably imposed by the policies of funding agencies and private foundations. The choice of these research directions becomes, therefore, linked to the expected financial profit of the pharmacological sponsors. "AIDS Business" was born on these grounds.

What are the tens of thousands of AIDS scientists throughout the world actually working on? Primarily, they work on the development of new antiviral substances and on problematic vaccines, i.e. products expected to raise considerable profits.

The new molecules resulting from this work will, probably, be as toxic as those currently used.

As for vaccines, that is another scary swindle.

Vaccination is designed to prevent an illness, by causing the manufacture of antibodies against an infectious microbe in a healthy individual.

Once vaccinated, a person becomes a carrier of antibodies that will protect him/her against any further attack by that same microbe.

Isn't that the definition of seropositivity?

Faced with this dilemma, scientists have circumvented the problem. Instead of wasting their time trying to design a highly problematic preventative vaccine (remember that HIV has never been properly isolated), they are concentrating their efforts on a "curative vaccine", a toned-down term for a new breed of medicines whose effectiveness will have more to do with magic incantations than science!

Actually, relying on the viral hypothesis of AIDS is a tragic mistake on two distinct grounds: on one hand, people, whether healthy or ill, are treated with highly toxic drugs; on the other hand, they are not treated to control the factors responsible for their condition. We have already indicated these factors (narcotics, malnutrition, transfusions, repeated infections, abuse of certain medicines…). They were well known and documented a long time before immunodeficiency was given a new name.

ASK YOURSELF KEY QUESTIONS

Y ou don't need to be a scientist to raise many most embarrassing, and so far unanswered questions:

- In Europe and in North America, a great majority of AIDS cases have been observed among males. Do you know any other infectious disease attacking 90% males and only 10% females?
- The "viral load" is defined as expressing the number of retroviral particles in patient's blood plasma. Have you ever seen a publication that directly demonstrates, by electron microscopy, retroviral particles in the blood plasma of patients allegedly presenting a high "viral load"?
- Millions of people have been terrorized by the announcement of their "seropositivity", presented to them as an HIV signature. Why was it practically never explained to these people that the tests used (Elisa or WB) only indicate the presence of high levels of antibodies, most frequently explainable by infectious diseases, heavy medical histories, or by previous blood transfusions, but are in no way the indicators of an active infectious process?
- Pictures of alleged "HIV", impressively colored and em-

TEN LIES ABOUT AIDS

bellished by computer graphics, are being published endlessly by magazines, worldwide. All these pictures were taken on complex laboratory cell culture samples, hyperstimulated by growth factors. Do you understand why not a single one of these "beautiful pictures" originates directly from one single AIDS patient?

- Anti-proteases are part of the HAART regimen. They have been demonstrated as being most active against Candida a. and against Pneumocystis c. How could you exclude the possibility that the favorable clinical effects frequently observed among HAART treated evolutive AIDS patients do not simply reflect favorable effects on the most frequent opportunistic infections, but do not, in any way, demonstrate a highly questionable anti-retroviral effect?
- Seropositive hemophiliacs, studied in the UK for many years, presented, until 1986, a fairly constant mortality rate. In 1987, their mortality suddenly jumped up by a factor ten, and more so in 1988, i.e. precisely at the time that very high doses of AZT started to be administered. How can you ignore the fact that this very sudden increase in mortality does not reflect frequently fatal, immunosuppressive effects of high dosages of AZT, and has probably nothing to do with the lethal effects of an alleged HIV infection?
- Well-known retroviruses from mice and chickens never kill the cells they infect. If the alleged "HIV" is a member of that retroviral family, how do you rationalize the hypothesis that HIV kills infected CD4 T-lymphocytes?
- Specificity of so-called molecular markers of HIV could have only been conclusively demonstrated if HIV had ever been successfully purified, i.e. separated from all cellular debris. Unfortunately, and as admitted by Luc Montagnier in 1996, this has never been achieved. Consequently, how can you understand the current reliance on HIV molecular markers such as p24, RT, etc,?
- Could you give us the name of one single AIDS patient that has been CURED by anti-retroviral drugs?

ASK YOURSELF KEY QUESTIONS

- If AIDS was really an heterosexually transmissible disease, how could you explain that, worldwide, the incidence of AIDS among prostitutes is extremely low, seropositivity being only observed among the sex workers that are also IV drug abusers?

- Could you provide the reference of one single scientific publication, published in the medical literature of the past 25 years, and that would have presented a conclusion reading something like: "We have isolated a so far unknown retrovirus and we provide scientific evidence showing that this virus is the cause of AIDS"?

- If AIDS was actually decimating the population of Africa, how can it be explained that this continent had a population of less than 400 million inhabitants at the beginning of the supposed epidemic, and that there were 682 million (excluding North Africa) at the beginning of 2005?

The number of embarrassing questions is endless, and any satisfactory answer to any of the 12 above listed questions would be carefully reviewed. We are afraid, however, that there is none. For some, there are "official ready-made replies"...but never the least supported proof. For others, the scientific community hides behind the fact that the phenomena caused by the virus, like the virus itself, are still misunderstood.

The alleged role of HIV in the causation of AIDS has taken the proportion of a quasi-religious dogma, and modern medicine may well represent a "New World Religion" as compellingly suggested by Olivier Clerc (See Olivier Clerc's book under References). If this is the case, other approaches to the HIV debate obviously have to be explored.

"HIV" has been by far the most researched virus in the history of microbiology! But what is the use of the colossal budgets spent on the study of this hypothetical microorganism, when after so many years so little satisfactory information has been obtained that would fit with the available epidemiological evidence?

HAPPILY, WE HAVE INTERNET!

Anti-establishment sites
In English:

- RETHINKING AIDS:
The official site of the Rethinking AIDS Group.
http://rethinkingaids.com

- VIRUS MYTH:
The site of Robert Laarhoven (Holland).
http://www.virusmyth.net/aids/

- AIDS MYTH (IRELAND):
http://www.aidsmyth.addr.com/index1.htm

TEN LIES ABOUT AIDS

- DUESBERG ON AIDS:

The site of Dr Peter Duesberg, leader of the protestors against the official thesis (USA)
http://www.duesberg.com

- ROBERTO GIRALDO:

(Also in Spanish)
Website of Dr. Roberto A. Giraldo, Infections and Tropical Diseases Specialist (USA)
http://robertogiraldo.com

- THE PERTH GROUP:

Website of the Perth Group, a group of scientists who contest the viral origin of AIDS, with a base of numerous pertinent articles and documents (Australia):
http://www.theperthgroup.com

- ALIVE AND WELL:

Website of Christine Maggiore, founder of the Alive and Well association which unites seropositive people who are nevertheless in perfect health (USA)
http://aliveandwell.org/

- TOXI-HEALTH INTERNATIONAL:

Website of Dr. Mohammed Ali Al-Bayati, particularly implicating corticoids in problems of immunodeficiency (USA).
http://www.toxi-health.com

- SUMERIA – THE IMMUNE SYSTEM (USA):

http://www.sumeria.net/aids.html

HAPPILY, WE HAVE INTERNET!

HEAL (HEALTH EDUCATION AIDS LIAISON):
Non-governmental USA organization
http://www.healaids.com

- HEAL TORONTO:
Canadian branch of HEAL
http://healtoronto.com

- ALTHEAL
Non-governmental British organization
http://www.altheal.org

- ANOTHERLOOK AT BREASTFEEDING AND HIV/AIDS:
Website dedicated to breastfeeding (USA)
http://www.anotherlook.org

- ACT UP SAN FRANCISCO:
Non-governmental organization (USA):
http://www.actupsf.com/

- ALBERTA REAPPRAISING AIDS SOCIETY:
Canadian non-governmental organization:
http://www.aras.ab.ca

In French:

- SIDA SANTÉ:
Not to be missed: regretfully, this is the only French language website devoted to the AIDS controversy. On the other hand, it is one of the best documented. It is thanks to the tireless efforts

of **Mark Griffiths,** dissident from the earliest time, seropositive and included in the category of "long term survivors", who died suddenly in the autumn of 2004, in circumstances that are not very clear. He had announced a short while earlier that he was going to take legal action against the firms manufacturing the HIV tests.

This site is currently accessible through the following two addresses:
http://www.sidasante.com
and *http://perso.wanadoo.fr/sidasante*

In German:

- RETHINKING AIDS DEUTSCHLAND:
http://www.rethinkingaids.de

- HEAL DEUTSCHLAND:
http://members.aol.com/nuejo61

- AIDS INFO NET:
http://aids-info.net/micha/hiv/aids/ain_index.htm

- AIDS KRITIK:
http://aids-kritik.de/

- VERTEIDIDUNG DER AIDS KRITIKER:
http://members.lol.li/twostone/aids.html

In Spanish:

- PLURAL-21
http://www.plural-21.org

HAPPILY, WE HAVE INTERNET!

- **FREE NEWS SALUD (ALSO IN CATALAN):**
http://www.free-news.org/index01.htm

In Italian:

- **LA VERITÀ SULL'AIDS:**
http://www.oikos.org/aids/it/default.htm

In Portuguese:

- **TEMAS ACTUAIS NA PROMOÇÃ DA SAÚDE (TAPS):**
http://www.taps.org.br/

To be added ...

- **UNAIDS (UNITED NATIONS PROGRAM FOR AIDS) :**
http://www.unaids.org/highband/index.html

- The report entitled: "Review of the AIDS epidemic – December 2004", from which certain tables have been reproduced in this book, has been founded on the site of **WHO (World Health Organization):**
http://www.who.int/

EPILOGUE

Yes, we have briefly analyzed the 10 biggest lies about AIDS. Admittedly, this book, initially written in French in 2005, has an obvious "French bias". It appeared, however, that the message of the "Ten major lies about AIDS" was likely to have a worldwide impact and, therefore, that an English translation was most desirable. The translation has been accompanied by extensive revision in many chapters, but the basic organization of the book remains the same as that of the original French version. Similarly to the original version, the text has been written, as much as possible, in a style that should be readable for the public at large, avoiding, therefore, accumulating innumerable specific references that are of interest only to the specialized scientists.

We do not want, however, to leave the reader on the totally negative and highly depressing notion of "Ten Lies", because, actually, there is considerable amount of hope in the "dissident" views regarding what is currently referred to as "AIDS".

To explain where such hopes originate from, emphasis should be placed, once more, on the fact that the HIV/AIDS hypothesis has created a devastating terror of a terrible epidemic, initially limited to the male homosexual community, then rapidly spreading to the entire world population. This terror was entirely based on the hypothetical spread of a supposedly lethal retrovirus.

However, in experimental pathology, leukemias and cancers caused by retroviruses in certain animals are **not curable**, by any medication, and cannot be prevented by any vaccine.

In other words, if it had been proved, scientifically, that AIDS was indeed caused by a retrovirus, this "discovery" would have been very bad news! **Fortunately**, a causal relationship between AIDS and a retrovirus has never been demonstrated.

Historically, there are many examples in medical science confirming the basic concept of Louis Pasteur, and according to which the precise identification of the causal agent of an infectious illness is a decisive step towards finding effective prevention or therapy.

However, no retrovirus has ever been found responsible for any human pathology. In particular, twenty years of intensive research (from 1960 to 1980) was not able to establish the least evidence that a retrovirus caused human cancer.

Linking a given microorganism to the cause of an illness is classically analyzed according to the four postulates defined by Robert Koch in 1884. These four postulates stress the necessity:

1) To isolate the suspected microbe from all patients;

2) To culture the microbe in the laboratory;

3) To transmit the disease, with the cultured microbe, to a susceptible laboratory animal; and

4) To repeat the successful isolation of the microbe from the newly infected animals.

None of these four postulates is verifiable in all the scientific literature relating to the HIV/AIDS dogma. Incidentally, several hundred chimpanzees were inoculated with the so-called HIV at the beginning of the 80s, in the CDC laboratories (Atlanta – USA), and they are progressively dying, not from AIDS but from ... old age!

EPILOGUE

AIDS is unquestionably a clinical reality, a "syndrome" with often-dramatic consequences. **But it is not an infectious disease.**

There is strictly no evidence that this illness is caused by a retrovirus like the ghostly "HIV", which has never been directly isolated from a single AIDS patient.

Neither is there any proof of the contagious nature of this illness, which entails the isolation of a microorganism, an operation that has never been achieved, even in patients with a so-called elevated "viral load". **(However, this does not change the most important recommendations regarding taking necessary precautions, including the use of a condom, to protect against true sexually transmissible diseases).**

Administering anti-retroviral "medicines" has never managed to cure one single patient. On the contrary, the high doses of toxic AZT given between 1987 and 1990 were probably responsible for a great number of deaths, in particular among hemophiliacs.

So, where is our message of hope originating?

Clearly, from a totally different understanding of the origin of AIDS.

How? By recognizing, from all the evidence, that acquired immunodeficiency syndrome is caused by a dangerous combination of toxic, behavioral, pharmacological and nutritional factors which have nothing to do with a hypothetical virus.

Exposing anybody to highly toxic drugs, or to medicines taken for far too long, or to chronic nutritional deficiencies, or simply to prolonged oxidative stress, shall, inevitably, lead to severe immunodeficiency with the resulting development of most serious opportunistic infections.

That this evidence has not been immediately recognized in 1981-1983 will probably remain one of darkest pages in the history of modern medicine.

It is direly urgent to drastically dissociate AIDS (a clinical evidence), from the so-called HIV (a totally elusive and ghostly virus).

It is also dramatically urgent to reassure healthy, heterosexual "seropositive" individuals that they do not have much to worry about and can live in peace (reference to J. Chin's book)!

TEN LIES ABOUT AIDS

Seen in this way, the preventative and therapeutic approaches to AIDS are radically different, simply because by abstaining from all poisonous drugs, by living under appropriate hygienic conditions and by eating a well balanced diet, the chances of efficient prevention and speedy recovery are considerable.

In sub-Saharan Africa, the provision of clean drinking water, good public hygiene, improved sanitary installations and adequate food are the most important factors necessary for the eradication of what is currently called African AIDS. Therefore the preventative and therapeutic approaches are drastically different in this region of the world, as the President of the Republic of South Africa, Mr Thabo Mbeki, wisely remarked in 2000.

In conclusion, we hope that by now our optimistic message is now clear for all our readers, and that the obvious directions to take for prevention and treatment are self-evident and, by the way, rather inexpensive!

Nevertheless, it will require considerable courage by scientists and health authorities to acknowledge the errors of the past.

Errare humanum est,
Sed perseverare diabolicum

(To err is human, but to persevere is diabolical)

REFERENCES

Although all the claims contained in this book are scientifically verifiable and documented, nobody is obliged to believe them on our words alone. For those who would wish to go further, here is a list of studies that have appeared in scientific publications, and support all that has been said previously.

All these articles are in English, which is the internationally accepted language of the scientific world today. Even French researchers publish their findings in the language of Shakespeare.

The studies listed hereafter are classified by subject and by date, in order to facilitate research. Certain can only be obtained by buying photocopies from the magazine. Thanks to the Internet, however, it is easy to at least find abstracts of the majority of these studies.

Later, we give a list of studies by "dissident" scientists and articles written by a few of the rare brave journalists (this list is a long way from being exhaustive), as well as a few books by French authors.

REFERENCES

CONVENTIONAL STUDIES

- **THE EXISTENCE OF HIV:**

- Barré-Sinoussi F. et al.: *"Isolation of a T-lymphotropic retrtovirus from a patient at risk for acquired deficiency syndrome (AIDS)."*, Science, 1983; 220, pages 868-871.

- Gallo, R. C. et al.: *"Isolation of human T-cell l Leukemia virus in acquired immunodeficiency syndrome (AIDS)."*, Science 220, 1983, pages 865-868.

- Baltimore, D.: *"Viral RNA-dependent DNA polymerase in virions of RNA tumor viruses."*, Nature 226, 1970, pages 1209-1211.

- Temin, H. M. and Mizutani, S.: *"RNA-dependent DNA polymerase in virions of Rous sarcoma virus."*, Nature 226, 1970, pages 1211-1213.

- Temin, H. M. (1985): *"Reverse transcription in the eukaryotic genome: retroviruses, pararetroviruses, retrotransposons and retrotranscripts"*, Molecular Biology and Evolution, volume 2, pages 455 to 468.

TEN LIES ABOUT AIDS

This article, written by Howard Temin, co-Nobel Prize winner (with David Baltimore) for medicine (for the discovery of reverse transcription) shows that this enzyme is not exclusive to retroviral activity, very much to the contrary.

-Varmus, H. : " *Reverse transcription.* ", *Scientific Am.* 257, 1987, pages 48-54.

- Hoxie et al. (1985): *"Persistent non-cytopathic infection of normal human T lymphocytes with AIDS-associated retrovirus"*, Science, volume 229, N° 4720 of 27th September 1985.
Showing that the famous "HIV" refuses to kill T lymphocytes in laboratory cultures.

- Smith et al (1993): *"Unexplained opportunistic infections and CD4+ T-lymphocytopenia without HIV infection. An investigation of cases in the United States"*, New England Journal of Medicine, volume 328, N°6, pages 373 to 379.
Study of atypical cases of immunodeficiency accompanied by opportunist infections in seronegative subjects.

- Gluschankof et al. (1997): *"Cell membranes vesicles are a major contaminant of gradient-enriched human immunodeficiency virus type 1 preparations"*, Virology, volume 230, N°1 of 31st March 1997.
Preparations destined for electron microscopic analysis are useless because they are heavily contaminated by cell debris.

- Bess et al. (1997): *Microvesicles are a source of contaminating cellular proteins found in purified HIV-1 preparations"*, Virology, volume 230, N°1 of 31st March 1997
The same conclusions as the previous study.

- **HOMOSEXUALITY:**

- Hayley (1980): *"Review of the physiological effects of amyl, butyl and isobutyl nitrites"*, Clinical Toxicology (unavailable).

- Gottlieb, G. J. et al.: *"A preliminary communication on extensively*

REFERENCES

disseminated Kaposi's sarcoma in young homosexual men." American Journal of Dermatopathy, 3, 1981, pages 111-114 .

- Marmor et al. (1982): *"Risk factors for Kaposi's sarcoma in homosexual men", The Lancet,* May 1982, pages 1083 to 1087..
Study carried out before it was claimed that AIDS had a viral origin.

- Jaffe et al. (1983): *"National case-study of Kaposi's sarcoma and pneumocyctis carinii pneumonia in homosexual men – Part 1: epidemiological results", Annals of Internal Medicine,* N°99, pages 145 to 151.
Table 1 of this book was taken from this study.

- Mavligit et al. (1984): *"Chronic immune stimulation by sperm alloantigens. Support for the hypothesis that spermatozoa induce immune dysregulation in homosexual males", Journal of American Medical Association,* volume 251, N°2 of 13th January 1984.
Sperm is a factor of immunodeficiency.

- Newell et al. (1985): *"Risk factor analysis among men referred for possible acquired immune deficiency syndrome", Preventive medicine,* volume 14, pages 81 to 91.
Correlation between the use of nitrites and Kaposi's sarcoma.

- Newell et al. (1985): *"Volatile nitrites: use and adverse effects related to the current epidemic of acquired immune deficiency syndrome", American Journal of Medicine,* N°78, pages 811 to 816.
Study showing how poppers invaded the homosexual milieu in the USA since 1976.

- Haverkos et al. (1985): *"Disease manifestation among homosexual men with acquired immune deficiency syndrome: a possible role of nitrites in Kaposi's sarcoma", Journal of Sexually Transmitted Diseases,* N°12, pages 203 to 208.

- Darrow et al. (1987): *"Risk factors for human immune deficiency virus (HIV) infections in homosexual men"*, American Journal of Public Health, volume 77, N°4, pages 479 to 483.

Study carried out in San Francisco showing the heavy drug use by homosexuals of this town as well as their high rate of infection of several sexually transmissible illnesses.

- Van Griensven et al. (1987): *"Risk factors and prevalence of HIV antibodies in homosexual men in Netherlands"*, American Journal of Epidemiology, volume 125, N°6, pages 1048 to 1057.

Study mainly showing the use of drugs in the Dutch homosexual milieu.

- Messiah et al. (1988): *"Risk factors for AIDS among homosexual men in France"*, European Journal of Epidemiology, N°4, pages 68-74

French study on the correlation between seropositivity and frequency of popper usage.

- Lifson et al. (1990): *"Kaposi's sarcoma in a cohort of homosexual and bisexual men. Epidemiology and analysis of cofactors"*, American Journal of Epidemiology, volume 131, N°2, pages 221 to 231.

Strong relationship between Kaposi's sarcoma and lifestyle of homosexuals.

- Seage et al. (1992): *"The relation between nitrite inhalants, unprotected anal intercourse and the risk of human immune deficiency virus infection"*, American Journal of Epidemiology, volume 135, pages 1 to 11.

Study carried out in Boston giving information on use of drugs by homosexuals in that city.

- Valentine et al. (1992): *"Anonymous questionnaire to assess consumption of prescribed and alternative medication and patterns of recreational drugs in a HIV population"*, AIDS Weekly, N°10, page 18.

Study carried out at St Mary's Hospital, London, showing the intensive use of drugs among English homosexuals and bisexuals.

REFERENCES

- Haverkos et al. (1994): *"Nitrite inhalants: history, epidemiology and possible links to AIDS"*, Environmental Health Perspectives, volume 102, N°10, pages 858 to 861.
Relation between AIDS and use of poppers.

- Woody et al. (2001): *"Substance use among men who have sex with men; comparison with a national household survey"*, Journal of Acquired Immune Deficiency Syndromes, volume 27, N°1, pages 86 to 90.
Risk of seropositivity due to drugs consumed by homosexuals in the United States.

- Vitinghoff et al. (2001): *"Cofactors for HIV disease progression in a cohort of homosexual and bisexual men"*, Journal of Acquired Immune Deficiency Syndromes, volume 27, N°3, pages 308 to 314.
Increased risk of death by AIDS due to the use of drugs in the homosexual milieu of San Francisco.

- Mansergh et al. (2001): *"The circuit party men's health survey: findings and implications for gay and bisexual men"*, American Journal of Public Health, volume 91, N°6, pages 953 to 958.
Drugs taken in San Francisco in the homosexual milieu.

- Colfax et al. (2001): *"Drug use and sexual risk behavior among gay and bisexual men who attend circuit: a venue-based comparison"*, Journal of Acquired Immune Deficiency Syndrome, volume 28, N°4, pages 373 to 379.
Drugs consumed during the big gay meetings.

- **DRUG ADDICTION:**

- Moss. (1987): *"AIDS and intravenous drug use: the real heterosexual epidemic"*, British Medical Journal, N°294, pages 389 to 390.
90% of seropositive prostitutes analyzed in this study were intravenous drug users.

- Rosenberg and Wiener (1988): *"Prostitutes and AIDS: a health department priority?"*, American Journal of Public Health, N°78, pages

418 to 423.

This article shows that seropositivity in prostitutes in Europe and North America is found almost exclusively in those who use drugs.

- Espinoza (1987): *"High prevalence of infection by hepatitis B and HIV in incarcerated French drug addicts"*, Gastro-entérologie clinique et biologique, N°11, pages 288 to 292.

French study showing that the symptoms relative to AIDS are common in seropositives and seronegatives in long-term drug addicts.

- Mientjes et al. (1991): *"Frequent injecting impairs lymphocyte reactivity in HIV-positive and HIV-negative drug users"*, AIDS, N°5, pages 35 to 41.

Study carried out on Dutch drug addicts. The lowered lymphocyte count corresponds to the number of drug injections, equally in seropositives and seronegatives.

- Mientjes et al. (1992): *"Increasing morbidity without rise in non-AIDS mortality among HIV-infected intravenous drug users in Amsterdam"*, AIDS, volume 6, N°2, pages 207 to 212.

Mortality rate of Amsterdam drug addicts is almost the same in seropositives and seronegatives.

- **HEMOPHILIA:**

- Darby et al. (1995): *"Mortality before and after HIV infection in the complete UK population of haemophiliacs"*, Nature, volume 377 of 7th September 1995

- **PROSTITUTION:**

- Smith and Smith. (1986): *"Lack of infection and condom use in licensed prostitutes"* – Letter published in The Lancet, Volume 13, N°2, of 13th December 1986, page 1392.

Results of studies carried out in Germany

REFERENCES

- Tirelli. (1987): *"HIV infection among female and male prostitutes"*, Announcement made at the 3rd International AIDS Conference
  This Italian researcher has published several studies showing the correlation between seropositivity and drug addiction.

- Modan et al. (1992): *"Prevalence of HIV antibodies in trans-sexual and female prostitutes"*, American Journal of Public Health, volume 82, N°4, pages 590 to 592.
  Study carried out in Israel. Absence of seropositivity in non-drug using prostitutes.

- Van Haastrecht et al. (1993): *"HIV prevalence and risk behavior among prostitutes and clients in Amsterdam: migrants at increased risk for HIV infection"*, Genitourinary Medicine, volume 69, N°4, pages 251 to 256.

- Potterat et al. (2004): *"Mortality in a long-term open cohort of women prostitutes "*, American Journal of Epidemiology, volume 159, pages 778 to 785.
  Huge study carried out in the United States over thirty-two years, showing that deaths due to AIDS are only found in prostitutes who use drugs.

- **MOTHER-CHILD TRANSMISSION:**

- Thiry, L. et al. (1985): *"Isolation of AIDS virus from cell-free breast milk from three healthy virus carriers."*, The Lancet, 2, 1985, pages 891-892.

- Blanche et al. (1989): *"A prospective study of infants born to women seropositive for human immune deficiency virus type 1. HIV infection in newborns French Collaborative Study Group"*, New England Journal of Medicine, volume 320, N°25 of 22nd June 1989, pages 1643 to 1648.
  Study carried out at the Immunology and Hematology Unit of the Necker Hospital in Paris, referred to in the text.

TEN LIES ABOUT AIDS

- European Study (1991): *"Children born to women with HIV-1 infection: natural history and risk of transmission"*, The Lancet, volume 237, N°8736 of 2nd February 1991, pages 253 to 260

- Blanche et al. (1987): *"Relation of the course of HIV infection in children to the severity of the disease in their mothers at delivery"*, New England Journal of Medicine, N°330, pages 308 to 312.

- **HETEROSEXUAL TRANSMISSION:**

- Padian et al. (1997): *"Heterosexual transmission of human immune deficiency virus in northern California: results from a ten-year study"*, American Journal of Epidemiology, volume 146, N°4, pages 350 to 357.

This study, spread over ten years, shows that the evaluated risk of a man "infecting" a woman is 0.09% by sexual contact, and that the reverse is still eight times less probable.

- Chin, James. (2007): *"The AIDS pandemic. The collision of epidemiology with political correctness."*, Radcliffe Publishing Ltd, Oxon, UK, 2007.

- **MEDICAL PROFESSIONS AND LABORATORIES:**

- Weiss et al. (1988): *"Risk of human immune deficiency virus (HIV-1) infection among laboratory workers"*, Science, N°239, pages 68 to 71.

Showing that laboratory workers are spared by AIDS.

- **TOXICITY OF ANTIVIRALS:**

- Richman et al. (1987): *"The toxicity of azidothymidine (AZT) in the treatment of patients with AIDS and AIDS-related complex. A double-blind, placebo-controlled trial"*, New England Journal of Medicine, volume 317, N°4, pages 192 to 197.

- Kolata (1987): *"Imminent marketing of AZT raises problems - Marrow suppression hampers AZT use in AIDS victims"*, Science, N°235, pages 1462 to 1463.

REFERENCES

- Dournon et al. (1988): *"Effects of zidovudine in 365 consecutive patients with AIDS or AIDS-related complex"*, The Lancet of 3rd December 1988, pages 1297 to 1302.
French study conducted at Claude-Bernard Hospital (France) showing that AZT kills lymphocytes.

- Clotet et al. (1989): *"Toxicity of zidovudine (AZT) in patients with AIDS"* – Communication during the 5th International Conference on AIDS.

- Van Leeuven et al. (1990): *"Failure to maintain high-dose treatment regimens during long-term use of zidovudine in patients with symptomatic human immune deficiency virus type 1 infection"*, Genitourinary Medicine, N°66, pages 418 to 422
Dutch study describing the toxicity of AZT in relation to the blood and the bone marrow.

- Chariot et al. (1991): *"Partial cytochrome c-oxidase deficiency and cytoplasmic bodies in patients with zidovudine myopathy"*, Neuromuscular Disorders, volume 1, N°5, pages 1048 to 1057.
The toxicity of AZT for the cellular mitochondria.

- Lewis and Dalakas (1995): *"Mitochondrial toxicity of antiviral drugs"*, Nature Medicine, volume 1, N°5.

- Grossman et al. (1997): *"Hepatotoxicity of an HIV protease inhibitor in dogs and rats"*, Toxicology and Applied Pharmacology, volume 146, N°1.

- Lo et al. (1998): *"Buffalo hump in men with HIV-1 infection"*, The Lancet, volume 351, N°9106 of 21st March 1998

- Wise and Reid. (2002): *"Neuropsychiatric complications of nevirapine treatment"*, British Medical Journal of 13th April 2002.
The damage caused by nevirapine to the central nervous system.

TEN LIES ABOUT AIDS

- **THE VIRAL LOAD:**

- Collective (2000): *"Human immune deficiency virus type 1 RNA level and CD4 count as prognostic markers and surrogate end points: a meta-analysis."*, AIDS Research and Human Retroviruses, volume 16, N°12, pages 1123 to 1133.

This analysis of 96 studies shows the lack of specificity and sensibility of the PCR technique in the diagnosis of AIDS.

- **EPIDEMIOLOGY:**

- Schopper et al. (1988): *"Sexual behaviors relevant to HIV transmission in a rural African population"*, Social Science and Medicine, volume 37, N°3, pages 401 to 412.

African sexual practices are comparable to those of Western countries.

- Dwyer (2002): *"President Mbeki might have a case on rethinking AIDS"* – Letter appearing in the *British Medical Journal* of 26th January 2002

Where the question of the surprisingly low rate of seropositivity in South African prisons is examined.

- Gisselquist et al. (2002): *"HIV infections in sub-Saharan Africa not explained by sexual or vertical transmission."*, International Journal of STD and AIDS, volume 13, N°10, pages 657 to 666.

Explanation of the false African "epidemic".

REFERENCES

STUDIES BY "DISSIDENTS"

- **BOOKS COVERING THE INCONSISTENCIES OF THE HIV/AIDS PARADIGM**

- Duesberg, P.: *"Inventing the AIDS virus."*, Regnery Publishing, Inc, Washington DC, 1996.

- Hodgkinson, N.: *"AIDS – The failure of contemporary science."*, Fourth Estate Ltd, London, 1996.

- Shenton, Joan.: *"Positively False – Exposing the myths around HIV and AIDS."*, Publ. by I. B. Tauris & Co. Ltd, London, 1998.

- Fiala, C.: *"Lieben wir gefaehrlich?"* (in German – Do we love dangerously?), 1999, Deuticke Verlag, Vienna.

- Brink, A.: *"Debating AZT – Mbeki and the AIDS drug controversy."*, Publ. by Open books, Pietermaritzburg, SA, 2000.

- Roussez, J-Cl. : " *Sida – Supercherie scientifique et arnaque humanitaire* " (in French), Marco Pietteur, publ., Embourg (Belgium), 2004.

- de Harven E. and Roussez, J-Cl. : " *Les dix plus gros mensonges sur le sida* " (in French), Dangles, publ., 45800 St-Jean-de-Braye (France), 2005.

- Farber. C.: *"Serious adverse events – An uncensored history of AIDS."*, Melville House Publ., Hoboken, NJ, 2006.

- Culshaw, R.: *"Science Sold Out – Does HIV really cause AIDS?"*, North Atlantic Books' Publ., Berkeley CA, 2007.

- Bauer, H. H.: *"The origin, persistence and failings of HIV/AIDS theory."*, McFarland & Cy, Inc., Publ., Jefferson, NC, 2007.

. **DRUGS:**

- Duesberg, P. (1991): *"AIDS acquired by drug consumption and other non-contagious risk factors"*, Pharmacology and Therapeutics, volume 55, pages 201 to 277.

A very detailed article on different drugs and their implication in AIDS. Available on the Internet website of Peter Duesberg.

- Duesberg, P. (1992): *"The role of drugs in the origin of AIDS"*, Biomedicine and Pharmacotherapy, N°46, pages 3 to 15.

- Duesberg, P., Koehnlein, C. and Rasnick, D (2003): *"Chemical bases of various AIDS epidemics: recreational drugs, anti-viral chemotherapy and malnutrition"*, Journal of Biosciences, volume 28, N°4 of June 2003, pages 383-412.

- Papadopulos, E. et al (1992): *"Kaposi's sarcoma and HIV"*, Medical Hypotheses, N°39, pages 22 to 29.

Demonstration of the responsibility of poppers in the appearance of Kaposi's sarcoma.

- **HEMOPHILIACS:**

- Papadopulos, E. et al (1995): *"Factor VIII, HIV and AIDS in hemophiliacs: an analysis of their relationship"* – Published in Genetica,

REFERENCES

volume 95 of March 1995, pages 25 to 50.
Available on the Internet website of Peter Duesberg:
http://www.duesberg.com/books/ephemophilia.html

-Duesberg, P. (1995): *"Foreign-protein-mediated immunodeficiency in hemophiliacs with and without HIV"* – Published in *Genetica*, volume 95, pages 51 to 70.

- **TESTS AND VIRAL LOAD:**

- Papadopulos, E. et al. (1993): *"Is a positive Western Blot proof of HIV infection?"* – Appeared in *Biotechnology*, volume 11 of June 1993.
Available at:
http://www.virusmyth.net/aids/data/epwbtest.htm

- Giraldo, R.: *"Everyone reacts positive on the Elisa test for HIV."*, *Continuum Magazine*, 5, 1988 (5):8-11

- Irwin, M. (2001): *"False positive viral load: what are we measuring?"*
Available at:
http://www.virusmyth.net/aids/data/niloads.htm

- **STRESS:**

- Irwin, M. (2002): *"AIDS and voodoo witchcraft.."*
Available at:
http://www.virusmyth.com

- **EPIDEMIOLOGY:**

- Stewart, G. T. (1989): *"Uncertainties about AIDS and HIV."*, The Lancet 336, 1989, 1325.

- Stewart, G. T. (1993): *"Errors in predictions of the incidence and distribution of AIDS."*, The Lancet 341, 1993, 898.

- Stewart, G. T. (1995): *"The epidemiology and transmission of AIDS."*, Genetica 95, 1995, 173.

- Stewart, G. T. et al. (2000): *"The Durban declaration is not accepted by all."*, Nature 407, 2000, 286.

- Geshekter, Ch (1999): *"A critical reappraisal of African AIDS research and western sexual stereotypes."*
Available at:
http://www.virusmyth.net/aids/data/cgstereotypes.htm

- Deru, M. (2001): *"AIDS in Africa – An on-the-spot experiment in Tanzania."*
Available at:
http://www.sidasante.com/deru/krynen.htm

- Fiala, C. (2003): *"Update in Uganda"* – Presentation made at the European Parliament in Brussels, 8th December 2003.
Available at:
http://www.altheal.org/statistics.fiala.hmt

- Girodian, M. (2005): *"Politically motivated disease causation. The biggest epidemic of all."*
This epidemiological study, written in May 2005, has been refused publication by every publication the author has addressed it to (that is sadly the general case). Nevertheless, it can be found at:
http://www.thenhf.com/articles_117.htm

- **RETROVIRUSES:**
- de Harven, E. and Friend, C. (1958): *"Electron Microscope study of a cell-free induced leukemia of the mouse : a preliminary report."*, Jour. Biophys. Biochem. Cytol., 4, 1958, 151-15.

- de Harven, E. (1965): *"Viremia in Friend murine leukemia : the electron microscope approach of the problem."*, Pathologie-Biologie (Paris), 13, 1965, 125-134.
This publication contains electron microscope pictures demonstrating very highly purified retroviruses isolated from the blood of leukemic mice (reproduced in *Continuum Magazine*,

REFERENCES

1997, and in www.virusmyth.com).

- de Harven, E. (1965): *"Remarks on Viruses, Leukemia and Electron Microscopy."*, The Wistar Institute monograph n° 4 (Philadelphia),1965, 147-156.

- de Harven, E. (1974): *"Remarks on the ultrastructure of type A, B, and C virus particles."*, *Advances in virus research*, Academic Press, New York, 1974, 16, 223-264.

- Lanka, S. (1995): *"HIV ; Reality or Artefact ?"*, *Continuum Magazine*, April/May 1995, (posted in http://www.virusmyth.com)

- de Harven, E (1997): *"Pioneer deplores HIV."* Published in *Continuum Magazine*, volume 5 (winter 1997-1998), page 24.

- de Harven, E. (1999): *"Viral etiology of human cancer: a historical perspective."*, *Haematologia*, volume 84, pages 385 to 389. (posted in http://www.virusmyth.com).

- de Harven, E. (1998): *"Retroviruses: the recollections of an electron microscopist."*, *Reappraising AIDS* 6 (11), 1998, pages 4-7 (posted in http://www.virusmyth.com)

- Craven, B et al. (2005): *"The anomalous case of HIV/AIDS."* Appeared in *World Economics*, volume 6 (January-March 2005), page 119 to 133.

- **VARIOUS:**

- Papadopulos, E. et al.: *"Has Gallo proven the role of HIV in AIDS?"*
    Appeared in *Emergency Medicine*, volume 5, N°5
    Available at:
    http://www.virusmyth.net/aids/data/epgallo.htm

- Herron, R. (2001): *"Why are the NSC and CIA managing America's*

global campaign against AIDS?"
Available at:
http://www.virusmyth.net/aids/data/rhaids.htm

- Clerc. O. (2004): "*Modern Medicine: The New World Religion. How beliefs secretly influence medical dogmas and practices.*", Personhood Press, Fawnskin CA, 2004.

REFERENCES

ARTICLES BY JOURNALISTS

- Tom Bethell (1994): *"AIDS and poppers."*
Article appeared in the magazine *Gay Men 360° Health*
Available at:
http://www.posh-uk.org.uk/gmh/gmh_poppers_tbethell. html

- Bryan Ellison (1994): *"The secret history of HIV."*
Article published in the magazine *Rethinking AIDS*, volume 1, N°9, of January-February 1994

- Gary Null (1995): *"HIV equals AIDS and other myths of the AIDS war."*
Article appeared in *Penthouse Magazine* of December 1995. Can be downloaded at:
http://www.sumeria.net/aids/null2.html

- Paul Philpott and Christine Johnson (1996): *"A viral load...of crap."*
Appeared in *Reappraising AIDS*, volume 4, N°1

- Djamel Tahi (1997): *"Interview with Luc Montagnier – Did Luc Montagnier discover HIV?"*
Interview published in *Continuum Magazine*, winter 1997 edition.

TEN LIES ABOUT AIDS

- Mark Gabrish Conlan (1998): *"Interview of Stefan Lanka, who challenges both mainstream and alternative AIDS views."*
    Appeared in *Zenger's Newsmagazine* of December 1998.

- Michael Verney-Elliott (1998): *"Virtual viral load tests – Seeing is believing – It's time to call their bluff."*
    Article appeared in *Continuum magazine*, Winter 1998-1999 edition.
    Available at:
    http://www.virusmyth.net/aids/data/mvetests.htm

- Christine Johnson (1996): *"Whose antibodies are they anyway."*
    Article appeared in *Continuum Magazine* of Sep/Oct 1996.

- Christine Johnson (2001): *"Viral load and the PCR – Why they can't be used to prove HIV infection."*
    Article appeared in *Continuum Magazine* of November 2001
    Available at:
    http://www.virusmyth.net/aids/data/chjtests.htm

- Neville Hodgkinson (2003): *"AIDS: viral catastrophe or scientific catastrophe?"*
    Article published in the *Journal of Scientific Exploration*, volume 17, N°1, pages 87 to 120.

- Liam Scheff ((2003): *"AIDS debate: the most controversial story you've never heard."*
    Article appeared in *Boston's Weekly Digest* of 7th May 2003.

- Rian Malan ((2003): *"Africa isn't dying of AIDS."*
    Article appeared in *The Spectator* in London in December 2003.

- Jean-Claude Roussez (2004): *" Les causes chimiques de l'immunodéficience. "(in French)*
    Article appeared in *Biocontact*, N°141 of November 2004.

REFERENCES

- Jean-Claude Roussez (2006): " *Sida : virus ou terrain affaibli ?* " (in French)
    Article appeared in *Biocontact*, N°163 of November 2006.

Made in the USA
Las Vegas, NV
15 November 2021